Dieting Can Ruin Your Health
The Japanese Alternative for Weight Loss

by
Hirotomo Ochi, Ph.D.

in collaboration with
Richard Bozulich

Ishi Press International
Mountain View

Published by
Ishi Press International
1400 N. Shoreline Blvd, Bldg A-7
Mountain View, CA 94043
U.S.A.

© Copyright 1989, Ishi Press International

ISBN 0-923891 02-1

Library of Congress Catalog Card Number : 89-80390

CREDITS

Cover Design: Ben Lizardi
South Pasadena

Interior Photographs: Takashi Kaizuka
Tokyo

Chef: Ritsuko Oyama
Tokyo

Editing: Elias Castillo, Tara Barmore and John Power

Typesetting and Layout: The Ishi Press, Inc.
Tokyo

Printing: Otowa Printing Company, Ltd.
Tokyo

First printing May, 1989
Printed in Japan

TABLE OF CONTENTS

Introduction

Japanese foods are gaining popularity and attention throughout the world. Not only are people becoming curious about things Japanese, people are also beginning to realize that the Japanese diet is the healthiest in the world. For example, tofu is a Japanese food that is eaten all over the world, not because of its taste — it is actually rather bland — but because it is recognized as a good source of protein, containing low amounts of saturated fats. Another example is sushi, raw fish on rice, which is eaten from the west coast to the east coast of the United States, in spite of the aversion most Americans have for raw fish.

These two items make up only a small part of the Japanese cuisine. There are almost 2,000 food items regularly eaten by Japanese. But it is not only the kind of foods eaten that give their diet its healthful benefits. It is also the balance of these ingredients in Japanese meals that makes the Japanese diet the perfect diet for health and longevity, and for maintaining a slim and fit body.

The purpose of Dr. Ochi's previous book, *East Meets West, Supernutrition From Japan,* was to introduce the Japanese diet to Americans, to show them how to incorporate this diet into their daily menus, and to explain why this diet promotes longevity, lowers the risk of heart disease, cancer, and the other diseases of middle age. In this book, his aim is to show specifically how and why this diet can help those who are obese or simply a few pounds overweight to achieve their ideal weight without literally starving themselves or risking their health, perhaps even their lives.

There are so many diet books on the market these days which promise their readers weight reduction. Unfortunately, no one can guarantee that everyone who is obese will lose weight, at least not without seriously jeopardizing their health. People become overweight for reasons that are too complex to afford easy solutions. But scientists report advances in this field daily.

In some people, obesity is clearly a disease that can be traced to a metabolic dysfunction. For these people, competent medical help from a qualified specialist is essential. Fortunately, this type of obesity is relatively rare.

Genetics clearly plays a role in obesity. Some people have a greater tendency to store fat than others, or they naturally maintain higher levels of fat in their bodies. Such people *can* successfully lose weight, but they must learn to accept their body type and not try to reduce to unreasonable levels.

Psychological factors are also important. People who are overweight and overeat are often castigated as being weak-willed, but recent studies have found that many of these people are almost powerless to control their cravings because of a combination of physiological and environmental factors. As one example, in the case of *carbohydrate-craving obesity*, the urge to eat excessive amounts of carbohydrates is a physiological problem triggered by an environmental factor, the length of the day. At the other end of the spectrum, there are those who suffer from *anorexia nervosa* and refuse to eat. This disease also has a physiological component in addition to psychological factors.

However, in the large majority of cases, ordinary obesity, commonly referred to as a 'middle-age spread', is caused by a combination of a sedentary life style and the high-calorie, high-fat diets that people who live in the Western industrialized societies eat. Our bodies cannot cope with the excessively high-fat diet that has become common in the last hundred years or so. This results not only in obesity, but also in heart disease, cancer, and other diseases of middle age. Obesity in third-world areas is extremely rare because people there eat diets that are low in fat, and they lead more active lives. This results in their energy intake roughly equaling their energy expenditure. But when these same people are uprooted from their natural environment and adopt Western dietary practices, they quickly become fat.

In the last 120 years, since Japan opened its doors to the western world, it has assimilated an enormous amount of western culture. But like the West, Japan is also an ancient and rich culture — its roots go back more than two thousand years — and the dynamism and inventiveness of its people are acknowledged the world over. Today, the pendulum is beginning to swing in the other direction, and Westerners are finding that there are a lot of things that Japan has to offer the West. One of these things is its food culture. Through a combination of trial and error, luck, and wisdom, the Japanese have come up with the perfect diet. It is a super diet, low in calories, yet high in nutrients, with an ideal ratio of fats, protein, and carbohydrates. The benefits of this diet for the Japanese population have been many. The Japanese have the longest lifespan in the world. They also have the lowest rates of death from heart disease and cancer in the industrialized world. But probably of most concern to the readers of this book is the fact that compared with all the other advanced industrialized countries, Japan has the lowest percentage by far of overweight people in the world.

Richard Bozulich
Tokyo, March, 1989

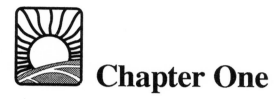

Chapter One

Dieting Can Ruin Your Health

Protein Deficiency Results in Death

Yumi Sato was obsessed with the fear of losing her slender figure.

Since 25, she had experienced problems maintaining her usual weight of 115 pounds, so Yumi was constantly going on and off diets. Still, by age 28, her weight had risen to 125 pounds.

She decided go on another diet, this time with a firm resolve not to break it until she reached 110 pounds. She selected salads, containing no starches or fats, as her main diet food. According to her reasoning, salads were best for dieting because they consisted of low-calorie vegetables which were 'healthy' — packed with vitamins and minerals. Her choice turned out to be deadly.

Yumi ate salads for breakfast, lunch, and dinner, occasionally adding some fruit and bits of other things. A few lapses notwithstanding, she followed this strict regimen for about three months, eventually reaching her desired weight.

Then one day she suddenly fainted while riding a train to work. She was rushed to a hospital, but by the time she had arrived in the emergency room she had recovered. Doctors, however, thought it best to run a series of tests. They found her condition essentially normal except for a slight irregularity in her heartbeat. To be on the safe side, they decided to admit her to the hospital and keep her under observation for a day or so.

High-Tech Medicine Fails

That evening and the next morning she ate regular, balanced hospital meals, but then in the afternoon she passed out again and was rushed to the emergency room. There, the doctors found she had developed a seriously irregular heartbeat. They immediately used a defibrillator and medications to try and restore a normal heartbeat. They were unsuccessful.

The emergency medical team did not give up. For the next 15 hours, doctors and nurses worked frantically to save her life. A pacemaker was even surgically implanted to stop Yumi's heart from beating jerkily and restore her normal heartbeat. Despite their best efforts and the use of the latest medical technology and medicines, the doctors were unable to save Yumi. Her heartbeat suddenly stopped completely and there was nothing the medical team could do to restore it.

An autopsy determined that Yumi's heart was normal except that microscopically its muscle fibers had decreased in size and protein content. The conclusion was astonishing — Yumi's salad diet had killed her. Without protein in her diet, her muscles had withered. Yumi's heart, which was also a muscle, had become too weak to support her life. Her irregular heartbeat was a dying tremor.

Beware of 'Revolutionary' or 'Breakthrough' Diets

Yumi's story is an extreme example of a possible result of compulsive dieting or following unbalanced diets recommended by self-styled nutritionists. Many of these diets are life-threatening if followed for a sustained period of time. Even if adhered to for short periods, some of them can be permanently detrimental to your health. Many diets nowadays are promoted with gimmicks or packaging which lead the unsuspecting user to believe that this is *the* one diet that will finally result in permanent weight loss. They are described as revolutionary or major breakthroughs. Some are written by quacks, others by well-meaning faddists. Many of these authors even have impressive medical credentials after their names. Ultimately, almost all of them fail.

If failure were the only drawback of these diets, they would be harmless. But they are not harmless: many are so nutritionally unbalanced they can kill.

At 1,000 Calories a Day
You Will Be Deficient in Nutrients

Make no mistake about it. When your daily diet contains only 1000 calories or less, as so many diet books recommend, it is impossible to get all the nutrients your body needs. We're not talking only about vitamins and minerals. These are important, but in order to stay healthy while dieting, it is vital to get a balanced supply of the three critical macro-nutrients: protein, fats, and carbohydrates.

Proteins are essential for the growth and repair of the body's tissue, such as the muscles. The best sources of protein are meat, poultry, fish, eggs, and soybeans. At least 12% of your daily caloric intake should be in protein.

Fat, as well as being a source of energy, is an important part of cell membranes, and is used for insulation and as a structural component. Fats are found mainly in meats and fish, dairy products, nuts, and seeds. Although fats are absolutely essential to good health, intake should be well below 30% of daily calories.

Carbohydrates are the starches and sugars. They provide a source of quick energy and are supplied in the diet by potatoes, bread, cereals, vegetables, and fruit. Carbohydrates should make up more than 60% of your daily calories.

Guaranteed Weight Loss, But . . .

Anyone will lose weight on a low-calorie diet which consists of 1000 calories a day or less. However, the loss in weight will not only be in fat, it will also be in muscle, or lean body mass. Not only will your skeletal muscles weaken but your heart — the body's most important muscle — will also lose tissue. When 15 obese patients, kept on a medically supervised 1,000-calorie-a-day diet for one year, were monitored, the average weight loss was 35 kg., but **25% of this weight loss was in muscle tissue!**

Even if you make sure your diet has adequate protein, muscle tissue, including that in your heart, will still be broken down if you eat fewer calories than you need for your daily activities.

Carbohydrates are the body's most direct source of energy. Having them in your diet reduces the potential of muscle loss, because the body doesn't need to break down muscle in order to produce energy. Fat stored in the body is also a source of energy, but under severe caloric restriction, the body breaks down both fat and muscle for energy.

Dieting Makes You Fatter

The usual pattern after a period of severe dieting is for caloric intake to increase to **above** normal pre-diet levels, resulting in weight gain. Unfortunately, this increase in weight comes mainly from fat (more precisely, *triglycerides*) filling up the fat cells, while the muscles regain their former size very slowly. So the dieter ends up with less muscle and more fat than before the diet was started.

The danger of severe dieting is that if it is continued long enough, lean-body mass, or muscle tissue, is permanently lost and cannot be restored. This fact has been verified in experiments with volunteers. Moreover, many survivors of prison camps suffer from this syndrome. Patients who have recovered from *anorexia nervosa* (a condition in which a person, most often a woman, is obsessed with losing weight and literally starves herself) also have far lower muscle mass than is normal. This is the reason why Yumi's heart stopped beating: it had lost critical protein that could not be restored.

Lose Fat, Not Muscle!

The aim of dieting should be to lose fat, not muscle. But almost all low-calorie, weight-loss diets will cause you to lose muscle and water (muscle is actually 80% water), as well as fat. This dehydrates and weakens you. The body wants to get back to its accustomed eating pattern. Finally, you overindulge and gain back the fat you lost. However, your muscles stay smaller. You diet again and repeat the same pattern. You are now firmly caught in the *yo-yo syndrome*. The longer you continue following these flawed diets the fatter you will get. The only way to break this vicious circle and to achieve the fit condition you desire is to adopt a nutritionally balanced diet and an active life style.

The Traditional Japanese Diet:
Weight Loss Coupled with High Nutrition

The yo-yo pattern can be broken. By following the eating patterns and exercise program presented in this book, you can lose weight, preserve your muscle size and tone, and achieve that slender, firm figure you've always wanted. The eating patterns are those followed by the Japanese, the most healthy, vigorous, and longest-lived people in the world.

The weight-loss plan described in the following chapters combines exercise and nutritious foods that are low in fat, low in calories, but rich in nutrients. Its goal is to permanently shed unnecessary fat — to shed it for the rest of your life.

Chapter Two

Why You Get Fat

The Human Body: An Efficient Fat-Storing Machine

The ability to store energy as fat was an important development in the evolution of animal metabolism. It enabled many species of animals, including humans, to live through times when food was in short supply or not available at all. This meant that those individuals who could store fat most efficiently had the best chance of surviving famines. But today, when food is so abundant, man's ability to efficiently store fat is the main cause of obesity.

On top of that, life in the affluent societies is relatively inactive. In rural areas, the search for and the production of food is a full-time, exhausting occupation; no one there can afford to be sedentary. Although food is available, it has to be obtained through hard physical labor. The conditions of life are such that there is no opportunity to get fat.

Physical Effort Is No Longer Necessary

In modern urban societies our work no longer requires physical effort. We drive to and from work, ride elevators up to our offices, and many of us sit at a desk all day. At home, we have all kinds of appliances to help us do our household chores. We no longer have to use muscular power to do such things as washing our clothes or sweeping the floor. We get our food by strolling through a super market, then wheeling a shopping cart to our car, unloading it and driving home. If we are too lazy to cook our own food, we can go to a restaurant and have it prepared and served to us.

Food is Interwoven into Our Social Lives

To complicate matters, even if we resolve to cut back on our dietary excesses, it is often almost impossible to do so without making ourselves appear a bit strange. Food has become an integral part of social intercourse. Almost all social interaction is carried out over food. A cup of coffee, laced with high-fat, high-calorie cream and sugar, is the minimum requisite. Social visits usually include food and drink, all of which are almost certain to be high in sugar, fats, and calories. To refuse is to be rude.

Quantity is not the only problem. The food eaten by man in our modern societies is very much different than that eaten by people who lived only a hundred years ago. Today our food contains more fat but less carbohydrate and fiber.

Our Metabolisms Cannot Cope with High-Fat Diets

There is no doubt that obesity is a disease caused by the high-fat diets and life styles found in the world's affluent societies. Our metabolisms simply are not adapted to the fat-rich diets the western world is able to afford.

In third-world countries, the lure of delicious, fat-rich western foods is irresistible. In these countries we can observe directly the effect of the transition from a traditional diet to a western diet. The result is a gradual increase in the number of fat people.

Studies in a number of third-world countries have found that more than 50% of people engaged in well-paying, sedentary jobs exceed their ideal weight, ranging from moderately overweight to obese. However, as the degree of prestige and the pay of the jobs decrease, so does the percentage of overweight people. And in the rural communities of these countries, where the populations still eat traditional diets, overweight people are extremely rare.

Rural Life versus Urban Life

Modern life, with its abundance and comfort, is like a great magnet, drawing the people who live in rural communities into the urban centers. They flock to the cities, even crossing international borders, to share in this wealth.

In today's sprawling cities, life is not physically demanding. It is no longer necessary to walk long distances to plow fields, to climb a tree to pick an apple or an orange, or to pump drinking water out of wells to quench your thirst. In the city delicious, sugary, canned soft drinks or 'fruit' drinks are available just by slipping a coin into a vending machine. Instead of pure water, we now get excess calories because even a canned 'fruit' drink is usually just flavored water and sugar.

Increased Calories Result in Increased Fatness

Back on the farm, foods could be cooked at a leisurely pace, using methods that were slower and healthier, such as boiling or baking. In the cities food is frequently cooked in oil. This is a tasty, fast, and efficient way of cooking, but it adds more than 100 calories to each dish cooked. This can result, in someone who eats like this daily, in the intake of over 100,000 excess calories a year. Indeed, studies have found that the average weight of a migrant worker who has worked in a city for five years is more than 10 pounds over what he weighed when he lived in a rural area.

What About Japan?

In contrast to other countries, however, Japan has a built-in, fail-safe defense against this invasion of Western foods: the Japanese devotion to their traditional diet.

In the most recent survey (1987) conducted by Japan's Health and Welfare Ministry, it was found that 60% of Japanese eat a well-balanced diet of only 2,053 calories a day. Fast and instant foods are eaten mainly by those in their late teens and twenties. These are primarily university students or young company employees, caught up in a fast-paced social life and too busy to eat properly. However, when these same people marry and settle into conventional family lives, their diets quickly revert to the traditional Japanese fare.

This lapse in healthy dietary practices among Japanese is confined mainly to a brief period in their youth. Through high school, Japanese youngsters eat home-cooked Japanese meals. The close-knit family structure, as well as the high cost of housing in land-poor Japan, ensures that college-age and young adults live at home. Consequently, they usually eat two home-cooked Japanese meals a day.

The Eating Patterns of America's Youth

Unfortunately, this is not the case in America. The dietary

practices of young people in the United States have taken a dangerous turn in the last 20 years, with ominous prospects for the future of American health. Recent surveys show that there are a greater percentage of overweight children than ever before. Additionally, the level of cholesterol in their blood has greatly risen over what it was years ago. Ordinarily, these are not problems associated with growing children. The change is linked to the high consumption of sugary, refined, and fried, high-fat, fast foods. When you also consider the increased time spent watching television or playing video-games, the findings of these surveys are not surprising. It makes one shudder to think what the state of American health will be in another 20 years when these same youngsters start to develop middle-age diseases.

A Preoccupation with Physical Appearance

While indulging in fries, hamburgers, fried onion rings, milk shakes, and sundaes, young Americans are extremely preoccupied with their physical appearance. The standards of beauty set by the fashion and advertising industry impress upon young women that 'thin is in'. As a result, adolescent girls perceive themselves as overweight and 65% of them want to lose weight. On the other hand, the image of the ideal man as big and strong causes adolescent boys to think of themselves as underweight, encouraging them to try to gain weight by overeating.

These contrasting standards have led to extreme dietary practices. Many men tend to overeat and overdrink, while many women are torn between the temptation of tasty, high-fat foods and the fear of getting fat. This can have quite disastrous health consequences for both sexes in middle age, predisposing them to cancer and heart disease. Women face a number of special risks, even in youth.

Women Who Refuse to Eat

An ever-increasing syndrome among some contemporary young women is *anorexia nervosa*. This is an eating disorder in which a young woman drastically reduces her intake of food because she believes she is overweight. She refuses to eat, or eats very little, eventually becoming dangerously emaciated. In general, it is very hard to get these women to resume normal eating habits partly because, in certain individuals, hunger can trigger the production of addictive natural opiates in the brain. Fortunately, this can usually be treated by using opiate blockers along with psychological therapy.

Most women, of course, do not go to such extremes, but due to their distorted perception of their weight, dieting among young girls and women who are not really overweight has become all too common. Such practices have been reported in girls as young as nine.

It Is Unnatural for Women to Be Thin

From a biological point of view, it is natural for women to be somewhat fatter than men. The reason is that fat is necessary for reproduction. If a woman's body fat falls below a certain level, she will stop menstruating and ovulating. This is no doubt nature's way of ensuring that both the woman and her child survive. Since carrying a child through birth requires up to 80,000 calories, plus up to 1,000 calories a day for lactation, the chances of a slim woman and her child surviving a famine would be nil. Consequently, nature has favored those persons who have a tendency to store fat. A woman whose total body mass consists of up to 25% fat is definitely not overweight. This level is actually ideal for good health and appearance.

Dire Health Consequences

What are the health consequences of young girls dieting? First, it stunts growth and delays puberty. Moreover, such restricted diets are nutritionally inadequate. This has many long-range health implications, the most striking one is that the woman puts herself at high-risk for developing osteoporosis, the loss of calcium from bone, in later life. Most frightening, however, is the fact that nutritionally inadequate diets have been shown to shorten life span.

You might agree that that's all pretty terrible, but inwardly you are thinking, "at least they aren't fat." That's right, they aren't fat *now*, but here is the catch: people who are calorie-restricted for long periods of time often have weight problems later in life. The reason this happens is instructive for all people considering dieting, so we will explain the mechanism in detail.

Why Dieters Regain the Weight They Lose

The *yo-yo syndrome* among dieters is notorious. It works like this. You go on a diet, succeed in losing weight, but then you gain it back again plus more than you started with. You go on another diet, and the same thing happens. You get fatter and fatter. Promoters of popular diets claim that by following their diets you will lose all your excess weight and keep it off. They urge you to go on their low-calorie diets, but they don't tell you why almost everyone who goes on such a diet later regains the weight they lost.

The 'Fat-Storing' Enzyme

In the fat tissue of the body there is an enzyme that plays an important role in the storage of fat. This enzyme is called *adipose tissue lipoprotein lipase.* Simply explained, the way this enzyme participates in the storage of fat is to break down fats (more accurately, triglycerides) in the blood stream into fatty acids at the wall of the fat cell. These fatty acids then pass into the fat cell. At the same time, glucose, the basic sugar into which most dietary carbohydrates are broken down in the intestines, is also taken into the fat cell. Here it is changed into another substance and combined with the fatty acids to form triglyceride. The more triglyceride in the fat cell, the larger it becomes and the fatter you get.

When you go on a low-calorie diet, the body reacts by increasing production of *adipose tissue liprotein lipase*. Then when food intake later returns to normal, the activity of this enzyme is much higher than *muscle tissue lipoprotein lipase*. This results in more triglycerides being broken down in the capillaries (very small blood vessels) of the fat tissue, reducing their availability to the muscle tissue. In other words, more fatty acids are taken up by fat cells than by the muscle cells.

People who have been on low-calorie diets for long periods of time have abnormally high levels of this enzyme. It is easy to understand why the ability to produce and maintain high levels of this enzyme during a food shortage has great survival value: after a famine, as soon as food becomes plentiful again, a person can quickly build up his fat stores to prepare for the next famine.

An Urge to Eat Sweets and Fatty Foods

At the same time dieters are literally starving themselves and these enzymes are at high levels, another phenomenon is taking place: they develop a ravenous desire for food. Moreover, their taste preferences change from what they had been before they were dieting, so that they desire fats and sweets. What this means is that there is a 'time bomb' ticking away in their bodies that will eventually go off. When they can no longer resist the craving for fats and sweets, they start eating again and caloric intake skyrockets. Then that enzyme, *adipose tissue lipoprotein lipase,* which has been increasing while they were dieting, will go into action, making them fatter than they ever were. Nutrients will be directed into the fat cells, with the result that the muscles in their bodies will get less nourishment. In the end, with smaller muscle mass and larger fat stores, their diet has ended in failure.

The Japanese Diet: A Safe Way to Lose Excess Fat

Whether you are obese or simply a few pounds over your ideal weight, very-low-calorie diets will usually aggravate your problem. One of the safest ways to lose that excess fat and keep it off is to turn to the kinds of foods the Japanese eat and follow a sensible eating plan and exercise program. By doing so, you can be sure that you will be getting the correct balance and adequate quantities of protein, fats, and carbohydrates, as well as all the vitamins and minerals necessary to keep your body functioning optimally.

Chapter Three

Japan: A Paradise for People Who Want to Lose Weight

90 Million Overweight People in the US

There are 30 million people living in the United States who are so overweight that they must reduce or their health will deteriorate. In addition, there are 60 million people who are moderately overweight and need to shed a few pounds. The shocking conclusion is that 90 million people, or 36%, of America's population needs to lower its weight. Other statistics show that the average American male is 25 pounds overweight and the average female is 29 pounds overweight. Little wonder, then, that radical dieting is so common in the United States.

America and the other industrialized Western nations have so many overweight people primarily because of the high-calorie, high-fat foods eaten there. Until this situation is changed, obesity will continue to be a serious problem in the West.

The Japanese Diet is Low in Calories

What and how much you eat is clearly related to physical

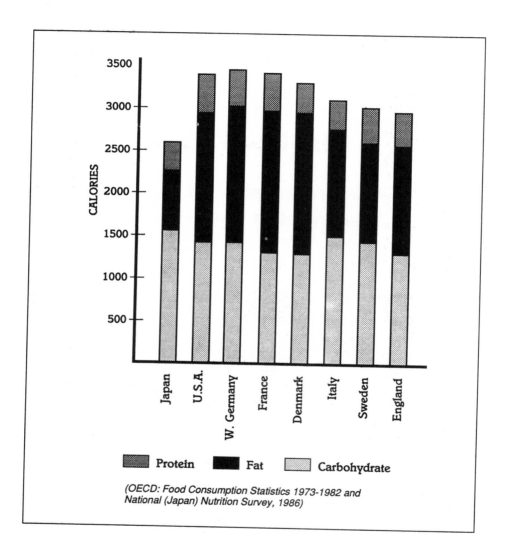

Chart 1
Caloric intake and the percentage of carbohydrates, protein, and fats in selected countries and Japan.

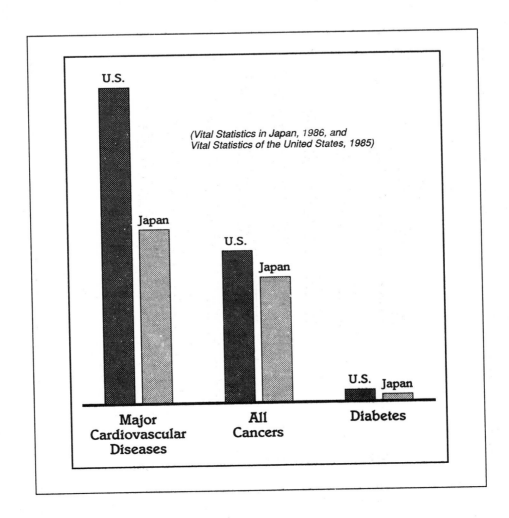

Chart 2
Comparison of death rates for heart disease, cancer, and
diabetes in the U.S. and Japan.

appearance as well as to health and longevity. In the advanced industrialized nations, food is so abundant that people tend to overeat. The people in most of these countries eat on average more than 3,000 calories a day (Chart 1). The people of West Germany, France, Holland, and the United States have the highest daily caloric intake at around 3,400 calories. By contrast, the Japanese eat only 2,600 calories, the lowest level among the world's industrialized countries.

High-Fat Diets Are Related to Obesity and Cancer

Not only are the diets of these countries high in calories, too much fat is also eaten. In the US, fat makes up 45% of the daily calories eaten. In Japan that figure is only 28%. Not only do high-fat diets predispose a person to obesity, they are also related to heart disease and various types of cancer. Statistics show that the death rate from cancer and heart disease is significantly lower in Japan than in the United States (see Chart 2).

There are also far fewer overweight people in Japan than in any of the world's other industrialized nations. Statistics published by Japan's Ministry of Health and Welfare show that the number of overweight people in Japan is just under 20%.

What is the reason for this great difference? The answer is not directly related to exercise. More Americans jog and participate in other aerobic exercises than Japanese. Ethnic background probably has little to do with this difference either. The Japanese who immigrate to the United States and adopt the same life styles and eating patterns as other Americans gain weight as easily as do native-born Americans.

When West Meets East

On the other hand, many Americans who live in Japan and adopt the Japanese diet lose all their excess weight. One example involves a couple who lived in Japan for over five years. When they first arrived the husband was more than 30 pounds and his wife about 18 pounds overweight. To economize (eating Western-style in Japan can be quite expensive) and also for convenience (their work required them to live in the countryside where Western foods are hard to come by), they shifted to eating Japanese-style meals.

Within two years their physical appearance changed dramatically. They both lost all their excess weight. The only major changes in their life style were their Japanese meals and increased walking due to a lack of convenient transportation.

Every day they would eat typical Japanese foods such as rice, miso soup, soybeans and soybean products, fresh vegetables, seaweed and fish. Their breakfasts were light, but their dinners were a bit heavy. In total they each ate about 2,000 calories a day.

Initially, this pair was a typical overweight American couple. Yet simply by switching to Japanese foods they were able to shed their unwanted pounds without severe dieting. After returning home they continued to eat Japanese foods to maintain their health and weight.

During their stay in Japan, they ate little beef. The main source of animal protein and fat was fish. Fish has more of the healthier unsaturated fats and less of the unhealthy saturated fats than beef.

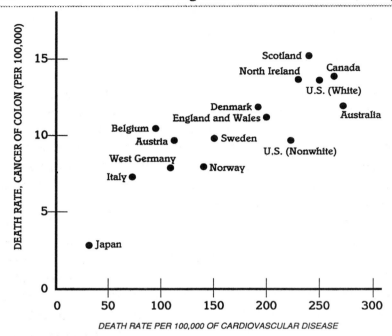

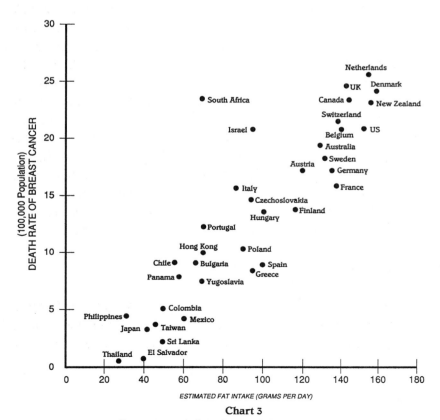

Chart 3

The apparent correlation between breast cancer, colon cancer,
arteriosclerotic heart disease and fat intake. A similar correlation exists

Japan Has Low Rates of Heart Disease, Colon and Breast Cancer

In the western nations, it is easy to overindulge in foods that have a high-fat content. This high daily intake of fat not only causes obesity but is also related to the high incidence of heart disease and cancer among the people of these nations (see Chart 3). Meanwhile, Japan, among the industrialized nations, has the lowest rates for colon and breast cancer and heart disease.

The death rates for stomach cancer and stroke are supposed to be high in Japan, but when we look at the statistics we find that the areas where these diseases are most prevalent are in the cold northeastern parts of the country. During winter, fresh vegetables are often not available, so the people there use salt as a preservative, relying on high-salt pickles for their vegetables. This high intake of salt causes blood pressure to rise, resulting in strokes. The high-salt pickles also create cancer-causing nitrosamines in the stomach, but a sufficient amount of vitamin C, usually obtained from *fresh* vegetables, which is able to neutralize these nitrosamines, is lacking in the diet during winter months. The result is a high rate of stomach cancer. However, rates for these diseases are not particularly high by international standards in central and western Japan, where salt consumption is lower than America and fresh vegetables are available throughout the year. *The diet presented in this book, however, is low in salt and high in vitamin C, so the problems described above will not arise.*

High-Fat Diets Result in Obesity

Many people do not understand that the human body is not suited to a high-fat diet. The natural consequence of such a diet is obesity, cancer, and heart disease. Reducing the level of fat consumption to 15%, or even 20%, of daily calories would, in one stroke, bring about a dramatic decrease in the incidence of these dreaded diseases.

However, we must emphasize that fat is essential to human nutrition, especially linoleic acid, a polyunsaturated fatty acid found in vegetable oils. Without it you would develop serious health problems. As in all things, moderation must be practiced. The problem is that western diets are *not* moderate. Affluence has led Americans and Europeans to forget the proper way to nourish their bodies.

One reason foods which are high in fat are greatly valued is that they taste good. In past centuries a high-fat diet was a symbol of wealth. In Europe, aristocrats and noblemen ate large amounts of meat, covered with fat-rich sauces and gravies. Creamy desserts would top off enormous meals of up to three main courses. Peasants, meanwhile, had to be content with only grain and an occasional meager serving of meat. Even today the pattern is the same: the poor countries of the world have low-fat diets, while the rich countries enjoy delicious meals high in fat (see Chart 3). For example, as the American economy grew, so did the consumption of fat by its population.

The Greatest Number
of Overweight People in History

Consider that in 1906 fat made up only 33% of daily calories in the average American household. Yet, by 1950 that figure had risen to 40%, and year by year it has increased to its present level of 45%. This rise occurred not only in the United States, but also in Western Europe. As fat intake increased, so did the number of overweight people. Never, in the history of the world, have there been so many overweight people.

Not Enough Fiber

In addition, people in the advanced countries don't eat enough carbohydrates. Moreover, the carbohydrates they do eat come mostly from highly-refined foods which contain very little fiber. But fiber is critical for weight control because it helps move food through the intestines quickly, reducing the calories and fat absorbed. It also gives a satisfying feeling of fullness that lasts long after a meal. Chapter Four discusses in more detail the way fiber, and in particular the special kinds of fiber in Japanese foods, helps to prevent obesity.

The Low-Fat, Low-Calorie, Diet of the Japanese

Look again at the figures for Japan in Chart 1. While only 2,600 calories are eaten each day, and fat makes up only 28% of these calories, carbohydrates makes up 60% of total calories, and protein makes up 13%. These are almost exactly the figures that most nutritionists recommend for good health and long life.

How Many Calories a Day?

The number of calories each person should eat every day depends on body size, daily physical activity, age, and sex. In order to lose weight, a dieter should eat a minimum of 13.5 calories per pound of body weight based on what his or her ideal weight is. This means the minimum a woman whose ideal weight is 100 pounds should eat is 1,350 calories a day, while a man, striving for an ideal weight of 170 pounds, should eat no less than about 2,300 calories. Chapter Ten explains more fully how you can calculate your total energy requirements so as to bring your caloric intake into balance with your energy expenditure.

When you are on a low-calorie diet, it is important that your protein and carbohydrate intake be high. The ideal weight-loss diet should be made up of about 15% protein, 15% to 20% fat, and the rest in complex carbohydrates.

Protein Is a Key Nutrient

This amount of protein — 15% of total calories eaten each day — is higher than normally recommended, but as Chapter One emphasized, protein is a very important macro-nutrient, especially if your caloric intake is low. It is needed for the growth, maintainence, and repair of body tissue. Without it, the body will feed on itself, cannibalizing its own muscle tissue, in order to sustain its minimal metabolism. There is no evidence that protein consumption at this level is harmful, as long as carbohydrate consumption is high. Another way of calculating your protein needs is based on your body weight. By this method, you should should eat 1/3 to 1/2 an ounce of protein for each pound of body weight. Unfortunately, if you are extremely overweight, this method doesn't work and you will end up eating far more protein than you really need.

Carbohydrate Intake Must Be High

It is important to emphasize that your daily intake of carbohydrates needs to be high because they are the body's main source of energy. Without sufficient carbohydrates, the body has to break down lean tissue to get this energy. A high-carbohydrate intake spares protein for its more important functions and prevents its breakdown. Moreover, sufficient carbohydrates prevent the loss of important electrolytes such as potassium, sodium, and magnesium.

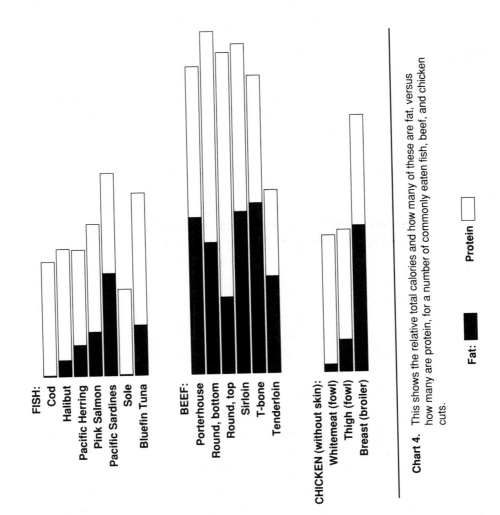

Chart 4. This shows the relative total calories and how many of these are fat, versus how many are protein, for a number of commonly eaten fish, beef, and chicken cuts.

Fat: ■   Protein □

Keeping That Slim Figure

The key to losing weight and keeping it off is to keep fat intake low. Even though you will be eating adequate amounts of animal protein in the diet presented in Chapter Eleven, you will not get a lot of fat. The animal protein will come from fish and chicken without skin. This kind of meat is lower in calories and has lower amounts of fats than beef and pork, making it most suited for a weight-loss diet. Furthermore, the fat in fish is healthier and evidence shows it protects against heart disease.

To achieve that slim, healthy body you've always longed for, your first step must be to cut down on your daily consumption of fat. It used to be thought that calories were all equal, whether they came from protein, fats, or carbohydrates, but it has been shown that fatty foods have the greatest tendency to be stored as fat by the body. Fatty foods are 18% more efficient than are carbohydrates in storing fat. Protein, by comparison, is only 4% more efficient at storing fat than carbohydrates. Therefore, the best way to lose weight permanently is to keep fat intake low, carbohydrate intake high, and eat only enough calories to supply energy for your daily activities.

The Japanese Diet: A Sure-Fire Way to Achieve Permanent Weight Loss

It is extremely hard to get a proper balance of protein, fat, and carbohydrates by eating western foods. Protein sources in these foods just have too much fat. For example, some cuts of beef — the kind marbled with fat — have almost equal amounts of fat and protein. Moreover, fat-rich gravies and sauces are an integral part of most meat dishes. You may think that low-fat or skim milk is a low-fat protein source. However, 100 grams of milk provides only about 3.5 grams of protein, a very small portion of the 50 to 70 grams of protein you need daily.

Fish: High in Protein, Low in Fat

Fish is high in protein and low in fat, especially when compared with the rich, fat-marbled, domesticated beef which Americans indulge in. Study Chart 4 and you will see how much protein you can get from fish and how little fat it contains compared to beef. Note also that fish has fewer calories than beef. Japan is among the highest of all nations in the consumption of fish. In certain areas people eat as much as 6 ounces a day on average. Japanese also eat beef, but not on a daily basis and nowhere near the quantity consumed each day by Americans.

Chicken is also low in fat, provided you cook it without the skin. For this reason, chicken is the other meat recommended for inclusion in your weight-loss diet. But the kind of fat you get from fish still makes it the preferred choice. Chart 4 also shows the protein-fat content of three of the best cuts of chicken.

Soybeans are Another Source of Protein

Another source of protein in the Japanese diet is soybeans and soybean products. The protein content of soybeans is legendary. Fortunately, these foods are available throughout the United States.

By eating fish and soybean products, the Japanese are able to ensure that their protein intake is high while their fat intake remains low, yet adequate. Following Japanese eating patterns will guarantee you a proper balance of protein and fat, making it very difficult and almost impossible for you to become fat.

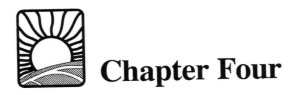

Chapter Four

The Traditional Japanese
Way of Eating

The Development of a
High-Protein, Low-Fat Diet

The modern Japanese diet is the product of more than two thousand years of evolution.

During those 20 centuries it went through many changes, incorporating other foods and cooking styles. Buddhism, which prohibited the eating of meat and fish, was a major influence. The result was the development of a large variety of nutritious, high-protein, vegetable-based dishes. Eventually, fish again became an acceptable part of the Japanese diet.

Moreover, the Japanese have always been willing to experiment with other cuisines. But only those dishes that proved to be exceptional, or of high nutritional value, were permanently incorporated into the Japanese diet.

The result is a diet that, if followed regularly along with the recommended exercise program, will not only strip all the excess fat off your body and strengthen your muscles, it will also reduce your risk of cancer, heart and other disease.

Weight Loss Without Hunger

Any diet that you follow to lose weight must fulfill the following four conditions:

- It must be low in calories
- It must be low in fat (about 15% to 20% of total calories)
- It must contain adequate protein, carbohydrates, fiber, vitamins, and minerals
- It must be satisfying

The traditional Japanese diet presented here fulfills each of these conditions. Not only that, epidemiological evidence indicates this diet can also lower your risk of cancer and heart disease as well as extend your life span. You get all this — weight loss, health, and longevity — without ever feeling hungry.

The Structure of a Japanese Meal

The basic Japanese meal is such that every needed nutrient is represented. It consists of a main dish, a side dish, and soup, as well as the staple, rice. The main dish supplies animal protein and fat, while the side dish consists of vegetables. The main vegetable source of protein comes from soybeans or soybean products like *tofu* (soybean curd) and *miso* (fermented soybean paste). Miso is usually served in the soup, and tofu can be an ingredient in either the main dish, the side dish, or the soup.

Tofu and miso are also important ingredients for providing the essential fatty acids. Rice, the staple of the Japanese

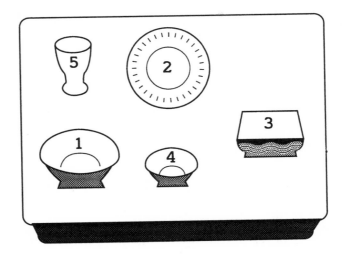

Chart 5.
The basic Japanese meal.: 1. rice, 2. the main dish, 3. the side dish,
4. soup, 5. green tea.

diet, provides the starch for energy and satiety. Finally, a cup of green tea, which supplies your body not only with liquids, but also a number of anti-oxidants such as vitamin C and E, rounds out the meal.

Rice: The Ideal Staple Food for Weight Loss

In the first three chapters we emphasized the importance of carbohydrates in any weight-loss diet. The main source of carbohydrates is usually the staple of the meal. In Western diets, bread is the staple, whereas in the Orient, the staple is rice. But when it comes to losing weight, rice is the ideal staple food. It is superior to bread on almost every point.

Rice Is Low in Calories

Looking at the calorie count, 100 grams of cooked brown rice comes to 153 calories, whereas 100 grams of bread may range from 240 to 265 calories, depending on the variety chosen.

Rice Fills the Stomach, So You Don't Overeat

Rice is also more filling than bread. This is because rice expands in your stomach, giving a sense of fullness. Consequently, you are less inclined to overeat.

Rice has one more important advantage with respect to losing weight. Bread is made from wheat flour which is ground up into a fine powder. This means that your stomach quickly digests the bread. Rice, on the other hand, comes in small kernels that must be chewed more carefully. In the stomach, it takes longer to digest than bread, so the feeling of fullness lasts much longer after you finish the meal. Moreover, since it takes longer to digest, the pancreas gets less stimulation, so less insulin is sent into the blood. High blood levels of insulin contribute to obesity by inhibiting the mobilization of fat from the fat cells.

One important point to remember in eating rice is that brown rice is more nutritious than white rice. Brown rice has all the vitamins that white rice loses in the milling process. This is especially important when you are on a low-calorie diet and every milligram of vitamins and minerals is crucial to the nutrient content of your meals.

The Main Dish

The main dish and the side dish of a Japanese meal are

called *o-kazu*. The main dish provides the animal protein while the side dish emphasizes vegetables.

Fish is the most important source of animal protein in the Japanese diet. It is usually eaten in some form or other at least once a day.

Fish: The Ideal Source of Protein

Fish is the most efficient way to get the protein that your body must have. It is also possible to get your protein requirements from vegetable sources, but this would require a much higher caloric intake, so there would be a greater possibility of weight gain.

Look at Chart 6 on the next page. Soybeans have the most protein of any vegetable product, but 100 calories of boiled dry soybeans give you only 9 grams of protein; 100 calories of tofu is about the same. However, 100 calories of most fish provide you with 15 to 20 grams, on average, of protein. From no other food source can you get so much protein with so few calories You should also compare these figures with the ones in Chart 4 on page 27.

Fish: High in Protein, but Low in Fat

Now compare the amount of fat that you get when you eat these different foods. In spite of all the hype that tofu has received as being a low-fat food, its fat content is quite high in relation to its protein content. Indeed, fish — and shellfish — are the most concentrated food sources of protein with the lowest fat content that money can buy.

Don't Forget, Fat Is a Necessary Nutrient

Don't misinterpret the above information data. It is

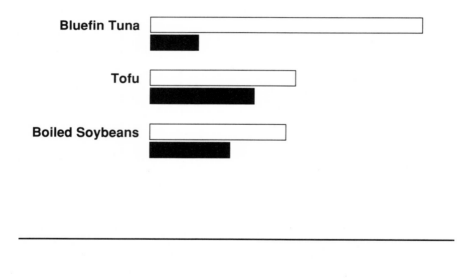

Chart 6.
Protein and fat content of boiled fresh and dried soybeans, tofu and tuna.

presented so that you can make a protein-versus-fat comparison. Soybeans and tofu are excellent foods and they provide many nutrients not found in fish. Fat is also a necessary nutrient, and the kind of fat you get from soybeans and tofu is less harmful to the body than the saturated fats you get from beef. As you will see, fish and soybean products make a nearly perfect combination.

The eating of animal protein in the West is always accompanied by a high intake of fat. This is a major reason why obesity is such a serious problem there. Making fish the main source of animal protein in your diet, and eating beef only occasionally, will bring your fat intake down to the ideal level of no more than 20% of your daily calories.

Chicken is also low in fat, provided that the skin is removed. One hundred grams of white chicken meat cooked without the skin has 24 grams of protein, but less than 1 gram of fat. In the weight-loss program presented in Chapter Eleven, we recommend that your meals alternate between fish and chicken.

Fat Plays an Important Role in the Body's Metabolism

If you are on a diet, your main enemy is fat. Yet fat plays an important role in the body's metabolism. It carries the fat-soluble vitamins like A and D and is the base for the structure of cell membranes. A shortage of fat in the diet is as bad as too much. It can result in a decreased immune response and even death.

Saturated Fats Raise Blood Cholesterol

When you think about the fat in your diet, you must think not only about the amount of fat, but also the kind of fat you are consuming. The fat from beef is mostly of the type containing saturated fats. These types of fats are solid at room temperature. They are also the fats responsible for high levels of cholesterol and triglycerides in the blood, which can lead to heart disease. This is one reason that you want to keep your intake of these fats low.

Polyunsaturated Fatty Acids Promote Cancer

High levels of the polyunsaturated fats (linoleic acid), contained in salad oils that are liquid at room temperature, have been implicated in the promotion of breast, colon and pancreatic cancers by inhibiting the immune response. Still, polyunsaturated fats are essential to good health. You just have to be careful not to consume too much of them.

Fish Fats Are the Best Fats

Fish contains a group of fatty acids known as *omega-3* fatty acids. These fatty acids have been shown to protect against heart disease and are not cancer-promoting. Since the Japanese eat a lot of fish, they have high levels of the omega-3 fatty acids in their blood. Americans, on the other hand, have almost none. This may be one of the reasons that the rates of deaths from heart disease and cancer in Japan are the lowest in the industrialized world. I wrote more fully about the omega-3 fatty acids in my previous book *East Meets West: Super Nutrition from Japan*. It is interesting to note that the main vegetable oils used by Japanese are soybean and rapeseed oil, both of which have significant amounts of omega-3 fatty acids.

The Japanese Diet Provides The Ideal Balance of Fats

It is necessary to emphasize, however, that a balance between the different kinds of fats is important. If you obtained your fats only from fish, your diet would have too great a quantity of omega-3 fatty acids and would be unbalanced. This could also lead to health problems. This is another strong point of the Japanese diet: not only is the intake of fats low, but the combination of the different kinds of fats that you get in the Japanese diet from fish and the oils in soybeans and soybean products like tofu is ideally balanced.

The Side Dishes

The Japanese eat a lot of vegetables in the soup and the main dish of the meal. However, the part of the meal where they are featured exclusively is in the side dishes.

Boiling is the most common method of preparing vegetables and it is called *o-hitashi* in Japanese. Boiling vegetables results in much lower calories than if the vegetables were cooked in oil. Of course, some vitamin C is lost, but Japanese also eat a lot of raw fruit, so vitamin C intake is high.

Seaweeds

Vegetables in the Japanese diet, also include vegetables from the ocean, namely seaweeds. A large variety of seaweeds are eaten by Japanese, but there are four that are used constantly. These are *kombu* (kelp), *nori* (laver), *wakame*, and *hijiki*. By eating vegetables from both the land and the sea, the Japanese get large amounts of minerals, vitamins, and fiber.

Japanese Food Is High in Calcium

It is the minerals from the vegetables and seaweed that are especially noteworthy. Traditional Japanese food includes all the minerals your body requires, especially that often hard-to-get mineral, calcium. This is good news for dieters. It means that you can get all the calcium you need without drinking milk, which many adults cannot digest, or eating other dairy products, which are loaded with saturated fats.

One green leafy vegetable, regularly eaten in Japanese meals, is *komatsuna*. It is one of the most concentrated sources of calcium you can get from land-based vegetables. One hundred grams of boiled *komatsuna* contain 210 mg of calcium. This is even better than milk which contains 100 mg of calcium per 100 grams. You can find this vegetable in many Japanese food stores. However, even if you can't, boiled leaves from the Japanese radish, *daikon*, available throughout the United States, contain 150 mg of calcium per 100 grams, and boiled turnip greens 160 mg per 100 grams.

Seaweed: The Most Concentrated Source of the Essential Minerals

The most concentrated source of calcium, as well as other minerals, is found in seaweed. *Hijiki* contains an incredible 1400 mg, *wakame* 900 mg, *kombu* 800 mg, and *nori* from 470 mg to 600 mg of calcium per 100 grams. And calcium is not the only mineral that they contain. Every mineral and trace element known to be necessary for human nutrition is present in abundant quantities in all of these four varieties of seaweeds. And you get them with almost zero calories. Adding them to each of your meals every day, as the Japanese do, will eliminate any worries you might have about getting your daily requirements of these all-important essential minerals. Fortunately, all of these products are available in food stores throughout the United States.

The Japanese Diet is High in Fiber

Fiber is another essential ingredient in a well-balanced diet. Although dietary fiber has no calories, it has many beneficial functions. It promotes the excretion of wastes and toxic substances from the body. There is evidence that fiber enhances the growth of beneficial bacteria in the intestines and controls the growth of the harmful ones. This is because certain kinds of fiber propel food through the colon at a fast rate and there is no time for food to putrefy. This action appears to defend against colon-cancer. Countries that have low-fiber diets generally have high rates of this kind of cancer.

Japanese meals are very high in fiber. High-fiber foods are found not only in the side dish, but also in the ingredients in the main dish, and even in the soup. And if you eat brown rice, it will also be a source of fiber.

Fiber is Important for Weight Loss

Dietary fiber is also important for weight loss. Highly refined foods are quickly digested and they stimulate the pancreas to produce a sudden surge of insulin. This over-reaction causes more insulin to be produced than the body can handle. The increase in insulin, in turn, causes the body to store fat. When the food you eat is high in fiber, digestion proceeds at a slower, steadier pace and the pancreas releases only as much insulin as is necessary.

The Kind of Fiber Is Important

There are many different kinds of dietary fiber, for example, cellulose, hemicellulose, lignin, pectin, and gums. They each have a different effect on digestion.

Cellulose, hemicellulose, and lignin are the structural parts of plants and cannot be digested by humans. Their main function in man is to increase fecal bulk, thereby preventing constipation.

The pectins and gums are the most effective with respect to losing weight. Not only do they increase the feeling of fullness, they also inhibit the absorption by the intestines of fats and sugars.

The Japanese Diet Has Many Kinds of Fiber

The Japanese diet is not only high in fiber, it is also high in precisely the fibers that will aid in weight loss. Seaweed, for example, contains a lot of gums such as *agar, alginic acid,* and *carrageenan* which slow down the rate of absorption of fats. This is why you should include seaweeds in your diet on a daily basis. It will make it that much easier for you to lose weight and keep it off.

Recent findings have shown that soybeans contain special kinds of dietary fibers, pectins and galactomannans, that reduce the amount of glucose and insulin in the blood. Not only that, experiments seem to indicate that these soybean fibers reduce fat (triglyceride) levels in the blood. These two facts indicate that eating whole soybeans or its fibrous residue like *o-kara* (see Chapter Fourteen), can have extremely beneficial effects on your efforts to lose weight.

The Japanese Diet Has Many High-Fiber Foods

Besides soybeans and seaweed, there are many other Japanese foods that are high in pectins and gums. The Japanese regularly eat a number of vegetables and fruits common in both Japan and America. Apples are especially high in pectin, as are oranges and carrots. These three foods are often eaten by Japanese, especially oranges. One of the best sources of pectin is oatmeal. It is pectin that gives oatmeal its characteristic texture after being cooked.

Pectin Reduces Hunger

A number of studies have also shown that hunger is reduced by eating raw fruits that contain pectin, such as apples. For this reason, an apple can make an ideal snack when you have a mid-afternoon craving for food.

Soup

A Japanese meal is always accompanied by soup, either a clear soup known as *suimono* or soup with miso. Japanese soups are low in calories and high in nutrition. They are made with a stock using the seaweed kombu (kelp) and sometimes other ingredients. The way stock is made is explained in Chapter Twelve. Once the stock is prepared, making the soup is simple, whether it is a clear soup or a miso soup. The ingredients are usually tofu and one or two other vegetables. Often, small pieces of fish or shell fish are added as the main ingredients for the soup. Japanese soups provide the finishing touch to the meal.

No Desserts

In the Japanese meal there is no place for desserts, and this is another reason why Japanese are rarely overweight. The nearest you will get to a dessert is a serving of fresh fruit.

Snacks: An Important Part
of Any Weight-Loss Plan

While desserts are not found in the Japanese meal, there is

nothing wrong with snacks, as long as they are of the right type. Snacks are actually an important part of a person's daily diet, especially for those who are dieting to lose weight. The problem is in selecting the right kind of snack, one that will supplement the nutritional value of your daily diet, yet not add excess calories. Including snacks in your diet relieves hunger and makes a diet easier to follow. In fact, eating small amounts throughout the day has been shown to be more effective in losing weight than eating the same amount of calories in one or two main meals. The Japanese diet is low in calories to begin with, so adding low-calorie snacks can give you the perfect weight-loss diet.

Sweet Potatoes: The Perfect Afternoon Snack

Fruits are often eaten as snacks by Japanese. Another favorite snack is sweet potatoes. Japanese sweet potatoes (satsuma imo) are one of the most nutritious snacks you can eat. They are extremely high in vitamin E (4.0 mg per 100 grams). The variety of sweet potatoes available in the United States is, in many ways, superior to Japanese sweet potatoes. For example, they have a higher vitamin E content. A 100-gram boiled or baked sweet potato comes to a bit less than 100 calories. A snack of one small sweet potato is a filling and satisfying way to relieve afternoon hunger pangs.

Carbohydrate-Craving Obesity

Some individuals, however, must be careful about snacks. There is a type of person who intends to eat a small snack, but then can't stop eating. These people can go through a whole box of cookies if it is sitting in front of them. Obesity caused by this type of behavior is known as *carbohydrate-craving obesity*. Recent studies have shown that this craving is one of many disorders brought on by the length of day: the shorter the day, the more these people crave carbohydrates. The cure is exposure to very bright light for about two hours a day. Lack of light is only one of the causes of excessive carbohydrate craving, but if you have such cravings, it is one of the things you might consider.

In any case, an **overindulgence** in snacks is one way to ruin your diet. Many people eat meals that are not particularly high in calories, but their snacking can add more than 1,000 calories to their daily diet. With the easy availability of soft drinks, candy, ice cream, and other sweets eaten for snacks, this is not at all surprising. An occasional treat is not forbidden, but if you are seriously dieting to lose weight, you must exercise some restraint and make sure that you are not exceeding your prescribed caloric intake.

A Word About Tea

Japanese not only serve green tea (*o-cha*) with every meal, they drink it throughout the day. This provides adequate water intake. You may not realize it, but you must drink a lot of water if you want to lose fat. Remember that water makes up 80% of muscle, so without it maintaining muscle size is difficult. Fat, on the other hand, contains very little water.

You don't necessarily have to drink Japanese tea to get your water. But next to pure water, Japanese tea is best. It is a tasty and enjoyable beverage and rich in a number of antioxidants, such as vitamins C and E, which slow down the aging process. Don't rely on getting your water from soft drinks or alcoholic beverages. Not only will these beverages increase your caloric intake, they will also increase your need for water.

There is nothing wrong with drinking coffee or other kinds of tea. Just be careful that the cream and sugar you add do not cause your calories to skyrocket beyond the maximum number you have allotted yourself for each day.

Chapter Five

What Is Your Body Type?

We all know people who can eat and eat and eat and still not gain weight, while other people seem to put on weight just by smelling food. How do we account for this? Common sense would tell us that those who eat a lot should gain weight. Yet it often happens that those who are dieting are putting on weight, while those who are stuffing themselves with those delicious fatty foods and sweets are thin as a rail. It really is unfair.

Two Ways the Body Handles Excess Calories

There are two ways in which the body handles excess calories. One way is that the body dissipates these calories as heat. The other way is that the body stores them as fat. Nearly everyone has the capacity to store fat and to dissipate excess energy as heat. But some people have a marked tendency to store fat.

Although your body may be the type that is prone to storing fat, this is no reason to be discouraged. A main reason for your fatness is your dietary style. There are many primitive tribes in the world whose populations have a predilection for storing fat. In their natural environment, none of them is obese. It is only when they come into contact with Western foods and a Western way of life that obesity becomes a real problem.

Your Weight Setpoint

The average person can overeat to some extent and not gain weight. His or her weight will fluctuate within a range of about 5 pounds or so. For example, a woman whose ideal weight is about 120 pounds might sometimes tip the scales at a high of 123 pounds, but on another occasion she might weigh as little as 118 pounds. To exceed her high weight might be just as hard for her as her low weight. This range of weight, beyond which it is hard to break through is called a person's *weight setpoint*. In one study, normal volunteers were fed double the amount of food necessary to maintain ideal weight for three weeks, yet they didn't gain weight. However, over the years, because of either a sedentary life style or overeating, or perhaps both, this setpoint gradually rises, resulting in a 'middle-age spread'.

Four Different Body Types

Everyone has a unique, genetically determined body type. Some people are naturally thin and others naturally stout. In general, they can be classified into the following four basic body types.

- **the fashion-model build** — small muscles and little fat on their bodies. They are usually tall and thin. This is the type that becomes a fashion model.
- **the athletic build** — large muscles but little fat. This type looks like a body builder. They have little subcutaneous fat, and muscles and veins are visible throughout their body. They have wide shoulders and narrow waists: the classical 'V'-shape build.
- **the stout build** — thick subcutaneous as well as visceral fat, along with large muscles. These individuals are

usually very powerful and, among men, are the type that becomes super-heavyweight wrestlers or weightlifters.

- **the roly-poly build** — large stores of subcutaneous and visceral fat but relatively small muscles. This body type has the most difficulty in reducing and often has some hormonal dysfunction.

Very few people are exclusively one of these types. Most people fall somewhere in between two adjacent types. They are a mixture of the fashion-model type and the athletic type, the athletic type and stout type, or the stout type and roly-poly type.

Setting Realistic Weight-Loss Goals

The above classifications are very important for setting weight-loss goals. The first thing you must do before embarking on any diet is to honestly evaluate yourself and determine your body type. One reason why so many diets fail is that people set unrealistic goals. They ignore their body type and diet unreasonably. This is especially true among women, and can lead to serious health problems.

Persisting in Unreasonable Diets Will Ruin Your Health

I'm sure everyone would agree that it would be ridiculous for a fashion-model type to try to develop the body of a pro-wrestler. Yet many women who diet are doing just this in reverse: their present and ideal weight for their body type might be 125 pounds, but they are trying to lose an additional 15 pounds to get that fashion-model shape. It's an impossible quest. Even if they succeed in attaining that weight, they will look drawn and haggard, and will lack zest and vigor. To persist in that quest will ruin their health.

Unfortunately, because of the dictates of the world of

fashion, many women who have a naturally large build, go on severe diets hoping to attain a fashion-model-type body. This is like a pro-wrestler trying to masquerade as a fashion model. He is doomed to failure.

Anyone Can Get Fat

All four of the above body types can have weight problems. Everyone will start to develop a middle-age spread from age 25 on if they eat high-fat, high-calorie diets and live sedentary lives. But those who are stout and tending toward the roly-poly build have to be especially careful. Those with these kinds of builds must start thinking about this problem while in their youth.

Fat-Cell Size and Fat-Cell Number

By the time most men or women have matured, they have accumulated a fixed number of fat cells in their bodies. In a normal 18 year old, these fat cells usually weigh about 0.4 micrograms on average. As this lean and fit teenager grows older, regularly overeats, and adopts a sedentary life style, his 'middle-age spread' is manifested by an increase in the size of his or her fat cells.

Dieting Can Increase the Number of Your Fat Cells

However, it is hypothesized that in certain individuals, overeating not only causes an increase in cell size, it also causes fat cells to multiply. A fat cell will first enlarge, then at some critical size it will divide into two, each cell returning to normal size. When this type of person goes on a crash diet to lose weight, the metabolic reaction mentioned in Chapter Two causes him to become ravenously hungry. He starts to overeat, fat-cell size increases, then these fat cells divide and increase in number. Now, in order for him to get back to his previous weight, he must reduce even more fat cells. Consequently, each succeeding diet this person goes on will be that much harder.

This type of obesity is rare, but those who are afflicted with it must be careful from youth on. The great tragedy is that they are also the very people who are most likely to go on very-low calorie diets. Yet these are the very diets that will aggravate their problem. The Japanese diet advocated in these pages is not guaranteed to cure obesity in persons who have a metabolic disorder, but at least it won't aggravate the problem the way other diets will. This type of person can lose weight, but his or her goal must be lower than those with simple middle-age spread.

Measuring Obesity

Intuitively, everyone knows the definition of being fat: it is simply having an excess amount of fat (adipose tissue) on your body. The man on the street and scientists will easily agree on this as a general definition. But scientists always try to define precisely the terms they use and, as a result, have come up with a number of precise definitions as well as formulas which range from those that can be used by anyone using a simple bathroom scale and ruler to those using complicated formulas whose terms require precise measurements by high-tech devices.

The simplest formula, one that needs only a scale and ruler, is to use height as a standard. The usual formula in pounds and inches is:

body weight (in pounds) =
{height(in inches) times 5} minus 198,

or, in symbols

$$BW_p = (5 \times H_i) - 198$$

Using this as a standard, someone who is 5 feet 5 inches tall should weigh about 127 pounds, while a person who is 6 feet tall should weigh about 162 pounds.

The problem with this formula is that it doesn't take into account differences in body types as well as sex. Some people have large frames and because of the differences in bone and muscle mass between men and women, this formula cannot be used as a reliable standard for judging if a person is overweight.

Height-Weight Tables

To overcome this problem, height-weight tables prepared by the Metropolitan Life Insurance Company have become the most-used standard to judge if a person is overweight. Table 1 gives various heights with the acceptable weight ranges in pounds for both men and women plus the average weight. If you have a small frame, you should be at the lower end of the acceptable range, while if you have a large frame you should be at the upper end.

Still Not Completely Accurate

But even these tables are not 100% accurate because they do not take into account the differences in muscle mass and fat between individuals. For example, many athletes have massive muscles but very little fat on their bodies. Since muscle tissue is denser, hence heavier, than fat, an athlete could easily exceed the acceptable weight range in this table and be judged obese. Yet, in reality, he or she would be lean and fit. On the other hand, a person with small muscles but with large stores of fat might fall within the acceptable weight range for his or her height.

Height	MEN Weight in pounds		WOMEN Weight in pounds	
	Ideal Range	Avrg.	Ideal Range	Avrg.
4'10"			92-119	102
4'11"			94-122	104
5'			96-125	107
5' 1"			99-128	110
5' 2"	112-141	123	102-131	113
5' 3"	115-144	127	105-134	116
5' 4"	118-148	130	108-138	120
5' 5"	121-152	133	111-142	123
5' 6"	124-156	136	114-146	128
5' 7"	128-161	140	118-150	132
5' 8"	132-166	145	122-154	136
5' 9"	136-170	149	126-158	140
5'10"	140-174	153	130-163	144
5'11"	144-179	158	134-168	148
6'	148-184	162	138-173	152
6' 1"	152-189	166		
6' 2"	156-194	171		
6' 3"	160-199	176		
6' 4"	164-204	181		

Table 1.
Weight-height tables for determining ideal weight.

Measuring the Fat Under Your Skin

A simple, but relatively accurate, measurement of how fat you are is to take skin-fold measurements. These measurements are usually taken with a measuring device at the triceps (back of the upper arm) and the subscapular region of the back, just above the waist. Through these measurements, it is possible to get a rough estimation of what percentage of your body mass is in fat. Of course, you don't really need to use these instruments since it is possible to tell if you have excessive fat on your body just by looking at yourself in the mirror and grabbing a handful of flab.

However, most people can determine their ideal weight by using Table 1. For example, if you are 5 feet 5 inches tall and have a small build, then your ideal weight should range from about 111 to 118 pounds. A medium build, from 118 to 128 pounds, and a large build, from 128 to 142 pounds. If you fall within the range for your body type, it is unlikely that you are fat.

Excessive Fat Equals Obesity

The percentage of body fat on a lean and fit man is about 15 to 18%. A women should have more, from 20 to 25%. If you have more, you should consider yourself overweight and to some degree obese.

Exercise Will Reduce Your Percentage of Body Fat

It is possible to reduce your percentage of body fat below these average levels through intense exercise and still retain muscle mass. Most male athletes are below the 10% level of body fat and female athletes below 15% body fat; some are far below these levels. This is true for athletes who practice aerobic as well as anaerobic exercise. Whether so little body fat is ultimately beneficial to your health in the long term is open to question. However, in a study of 5,398 female college graduates, half of whom were athletes and half of whom were not, it was found that the rates of breast cancer and cancer of the reproductive organs were significantly lower among those who had previously been athletes than among those who were not.

In order to illustrate the point that bodyweight is no indication of being overweight, look at the drawing on the next page of two hypothetical women who are 5 feet 5 inches tall. The one on the right has a large build and weighs 135 pounds. The one on the left has a small build and

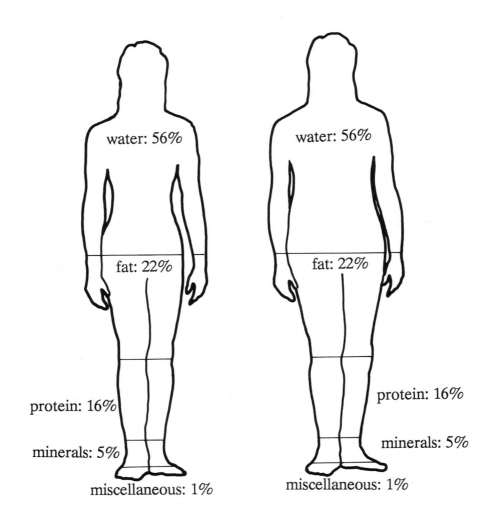

water: 56%

water: 56%

fat: 22%

fat: 22%

protein: 16%

protein: 16%

minerals: 5%

minerals: 5%

miscellaneous: 1%

miscellaneous: 1%

Two hypothetical women with the same percentage of body fat, protein, bone, and water. Although there is a 20-pound difference in body weight, each is of ideal weight.

weighs 115 pounds. However, both have body-fat percent-
ages of 22%, so neither can be considered fat, in spite of a
20-pound difference in weight. For this 135-pound woman
to get her weight down to match that of the 115-pound
women might be possible, but it could ruin her health.

The Aim of Dieting

The aim of dieting is *not* necessarily to become thin, but to
avoid becoming fat. Another, equally important aim, is to
promote health and to slow down the aging process. If you
fail to realize this point, even though you may lose some
weight, both your body and spirit will suffer. Of course,
weight and fat loss is possible, but you must set realistic
goals. For those individuals who are extremely obese or
who have been overweight for most of their adult lives,
reaching their 'ideal weight' may not be possible. Such persons have to lower their goals.

Maintainable Weight

There is a way that you can determine fairly accurately
what weight level is most realistic for you to maintain. It is
called your *maintainable weight* (MW). You can calculate
this weight by adding to your ideal weight (IW) two
pounds for every ten years that you have been obese, plus
2 pounds for every ten years you are over the age of 20,
plus 1 pound for every 10 pounds you are overweight.

For example, the 'maintainable weight' of a 5-foot 5-inch
woman whose ideal weight is 128 pounds, but is 40 years
old, has been obese since she was 15, and weighs 178
pounds would be:

$$MW = 128 + 2 \times 15/10 + 2 \times (40-20)/10 + (178-128)/10$$
$$= 128 + 3 + 4 + 5 = 140 \, pounds.$$

Similar formulas have been used successfully to accurately predict how much a person can reduce without subsequently regaining the weight lost.

The Great Advantage of the Japanese Diet

Whether your goal is to attain your ideal weight or your maintainable weight, the Japanese diet offers you the greatest chance of success. Foods used in this diet are, calorie for calorie, among the most nutrient-dense foods available. In other words, you don't have to eat a lot of calories to get your essential protein, vitamins and minerals. These foods are, moreover, low in fat.

The biggest advantage of the Japanese dieting plan presented in this book is that it is a total diet and exercise plan. It balances food intake with your energy output. By stimulating your muscles to grow through certain specialized exercises, you will 'burn off' your excess fat, and you will become slimmer and fitter than ever before.

Losing Weight Without Pain and Hunger

It is a misconception that dieting to lose weight requires an extreme reduction of food intake accompanied by pain and hunger. Such a diet is only a foolish activity that can ruin your health and shorten your life.

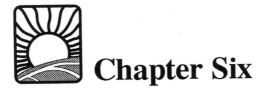 **Chapter Six**

Exercise and Losing Weight

Exercise Shrinks Your Fat Cells

Exercise is an important part of any weight loss program. The reason is not so much that it causes your body to burn more calories, but that it causes certain metabolic changes that make muscle tissue grow and fat cells shrink.

Fat Takes up More Room than Muscle

However, don't expect yourself to look like a muscular body builder. Getting that kind of body takes years of intense training. Moreover, because women have low levels of certain muscle-building hormones, large muscles are extremely difficult for them to obtain. What you can expect from the exercise program presented in this book is an increase in muscle tone and a slight increase in muscle mass with a sizeable decrease in fat stores. Even if you are able to exchange only five pounds of fat for the same weight in muscle, it will do wonders for your appearance because muscle is denser than fat, so it takes up less room. Your end result will be a firmer, more slender body.

Studies Show that Exercise Breaks Down Fat

Consider what exercise has been proven to do. In one 20-week study, overweight, sedentary subjects who continued to eat normally, engaged in an exercise program. This alone was able to cause significant reductions in fat mass, fat-cell weight, and subcutaneous skinfold measurements even though no significant reduction in weight resulted.

Fat Cells Resist Shrinkage

When lean, sedentary subjects engaged in the same exercise program, muscle size increased, but no fat loss resulted. This was interpreted to mean that there is a point after which fat cells resist reduction in size. When this point is reached, you have achieved your ideal weight.

Initial Fat Loss is High

Another study showed that obese persons who started on an exercise program initially had high levels of fat loss. After about three months their fat loss leveled off. In order for them to keep on losing fat the intensity of their exercise had to be increased. If you are able to reach this level, you could consider your weight-loss plan a success. Don't think, however, that you can afford to relax and stop exercising at this point.

If Exercise Stops, Fat Is Rapidly Regained

Other studies and experiments have shown that people lose the beneficial effects of exercise and rapidly regain their fat only 8 weeks after exercise stops. You must continue your exercise program to maintain your weight loss. This is especially true if you have had a problem with your weight in the past. However, once you have gotten yourself into shape, the level of exercise intensity need not be as great as when you were taking off the excess weight. A scaled-down workout schedule is enough to maintain your new body.

It's Hard to Reduce with Exercise Alone

Yet the effect of exercise on the number of calories burned is not as big as you might expect. While it is possible to reduce only by exercise, you will get the best results from both moderate exercise and moderate caloric restriction. The list below shows the number of calories you can expect to burn up doing some common types of exercise:

- **Jogging**: 100 calories every 9 minutes
- **Swimming**: 100 calories every 9 minutes
- **Aerobic dance**: 100 calories every 12 minutes
- **Weight training**: 100 calories every 13 minutes
- **Brisk walking**: 100 calories every 20 minutes

Exercise Cannot Keep up with Overeating

So even if you jog for one hour you will consume only 666 calories — the number of calories in a couple of snacks or in your favorite dessert. And if you are eating an average American diet of around 3,400 calories a day, assuming that the maintainence diet for a person of average height and build is only 2,000 calories, an hour of jogging still leaves you with a surplus of more than 700 calories each day.

Exercising and Dieting Must Go Hand in Hand

Of course, exercise, which uses energy, contributes to keeping your energy intake and energy expenditure in balance. But if you are overweight, the main reason exercise must go hand in hand with dieting in your weight-loss plan is that it causes important changes in your body's metabolism.

Lipoprotein Lipase Activity Is Decreased

The enzyme *adipose tissue lipoprotein lipase* was already discussed in Chapter Two. Experiments have shown that after vigorous exercise *lipoprotein lipase* activity in muscle tissue is increased up to ten times, while *adipose tissue lipoprotein lipase* activity in fat tissue is decreased by as much as 30%. These effects last for several hours after exercise. However, when you don't use your muscles triglycerides in the fat cells are not broken down. In other words, since the muscles do not use energy, there is no need to break down triglycerides. The result is that the fat cells keep growing and growing. In contrast, these same experiments demonstrated that this enzyme's activity in storing fat can be doubled by eating several heavy meals over the course of a day.

A sedentary life style also contributes to increased fat storage because when muscles are not used, they take up less glucose than they would if they were active. This makes more glucose available to the fat cells, so more triglycerides are synthesized. Consequently, your fat cells become larger and you get fatter.

The exercise program presented here will stimulate the growth of the major muscles in your body, maximizing the ability of your body to burn fat. Moreover, by eating the Japanese meals described in Chapter Eleven, you will get adequate nutrition so that there is no loss of muscle tissue. Instead, your muscles will grow, while your fat stores decrease. Finally, with the implementation plan presented here, you can be sure that the calories you eat and the calories you burn up through your daily activities will be in balance. The slight deficit in calories eaten is necessary in order for you to lose weight. With this diet you do not have to be hungry all the time. This makes this diet easy to follow and helps you avoid the yo-yo syndrome.

Exercise at Your Own Pace

The exercise routines presented here are not demanding. You do them at your own pace and not every day. Your workouts are geared to your own particular endurance levels and increase as you build up stamina. It is not necessary for you to exhaust yourself trying to burn up calories. The purpose of these exercises is not to burn up calories, but to stimulate muscles throughout your body to grow and to burn fat. In this way, your body's fat-storing metabolism is balanced. In other words, you do only enough to make sure that your muscles are stimulated and do not decrease in size. Moreover, you do not have to go to a gym if you don't want to. These exercises can be done in the privacy of your own home.

Aerobic Resistance Training

The exercise plan you will follow consists of a series of eight exercises using light dumbells that exercise every major muscle in your body. By doing these exercises non-stop, you give your cardiovascular system the exercise it requires. There are many advantages to this exercise routine:

It is completely safe. Everything you do is controlled; you don't make the sudden, jerky, or explosive movements that you might when playing sports. It is those types of movements that are the major cause of many sports-related injuries. You also have control over the amount of weight you use so that you don't strain yourself. Injury makes exercise difficult to do, in turn making it more likely that the injured person will become sedentary and lose the weight-reducing benefits of exercise.

It exercises all the major muscles in your body. This results in balanced development. In this way, every muscle in your body is helping you lose weight and increasing metabolic efficiency.

It doesn't take much time. These exercises can be completed in less than 15 minutes. And you don't do them every day. Three to four times a week is all that is necessary. Remember, recuperation is just as important in a training program as the exercises themselves.

It is convenient. You can do these exercises in your own home, rain or shine. There is no expensive equipment to purchase, nor need you pay to become a member of a training center. This makes it easier to exercise regularly.

It is easy to do. There are no complicated movements or techniques that you have to learn. All movements are completely natural.

Start Out Slowly

If you are out of shape, it is important that you start out slowly. Don't try to do the full routine the first time out. For your first session or for the first week you should just practice the proper form for these exercises. When you have mastered them, start out by doing about 5 repetitions of each exercise and gradually increase this number in subsequent workouts.

More Is Not Necessarily Better

As mentioned previously, undereating is just as bad as overeating. In the same way, both overexercising and underexercising are bad for the body. Some people believe falsely that overeating must be accompanied by intense exercise to use up the excess calories taken in, and that exercise is not advisable for those who habitually undereat. The truth is that *any* extreme can have negative effects on the body. Both undereating and overexercising can lead to health problems such as cardiac arrhythmias, while overeating and a sedentary life style lead to obesity and the diseases of middle age.

Moderation is the Key to Both Exercise and Eating

Therefore it is important to practice moderation in both eating and exercise. The aim is to find a balance between the number of calories eaten and the number of calories burned up in your daily activities. People who live long lives are usually moderately active and eat low-calorie diets. When their diets have analyzed, it has been found that they are nutritionally balanced and have caloric intake sufficient to maintain the activities of their daily lives. Needless to say, obesity is not a problem among these people.

Chapter Seven

The Exercise Program

This chapter introduces the eight basic exercises and comments on the best way to make use of them.

A word of caution. Before you start on this or any other exercise program, be sure to have a proper physical examination, including a heart and blood pressure check. If you have any problems, such as a bad back, do not engage in any kind of training program without the approval *and* supervision of a competent physician.

1. Stiff-Legged Bendover

Stand with the dumbbells at your side and your legs about
a foot apart. Keeping your legs straight with the dumbbells
hanging, take a deep breath and bend over slowly as far as
you can comfortably go, exhaling as you move. Straighten
up to the starting position, taking a deep breath. Perform
the required number of repetitions.

This exercise develops and strengthens the hamstring
muscles in the back of the legs and the muscles in the
small of the back.

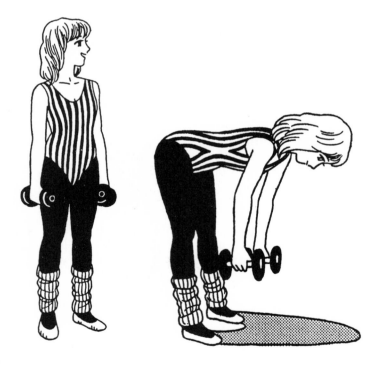

2. Bench Press

Lie down on a narrow bench. Bring the dumbbells up to your chest as shown in the drawing. From this position, take a deep breath and slowly push both dumbbells up toward the ceiling, gradually bringing them together as your arms straighten out. Exhale continuously as you straighten your arms. Take a deep breath as you lower the dumbbells slowly to the starting position. Repeat. This exercise strengthens the muscles in the chest, the back, the shoulders, and the arms.

If you do not have a bench conveniently available, you can do this exercise lying on the floor. However, you should lie on top of one or two pillows so that your chest is raised from about 6 inches to a foot off the floor. In this way, your elbows won't touch the floor in the starting position and you can maximize the stretch of your chest muscles.

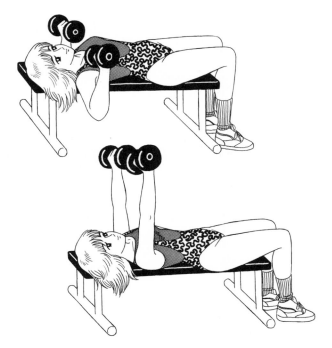

3. Toe Raises

Stand with your feet about a foot apart, holding on to something to maintain your balance if necessary. Take a deep breath. Rise up slowly on the balls of your feet, exhaling as you go up. Then lower yourself slowly, while taking a deep breath, so that you end up standing on your heels again. Repeat.

This exercise will strengthen the the muscles of your feet, ankles, and calves.

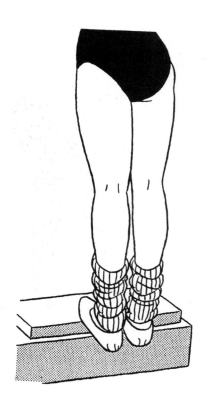
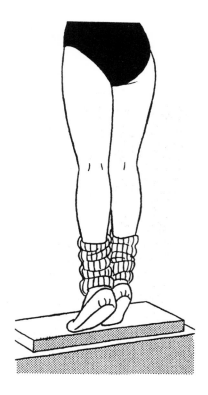

4. Bent-Over Rowing

Start in a bent-over position, legs slightly bent, feet about a foot and a half apart. While grasping the weights, let your arms hang. Take a deep breath, then pull the dumbbells slowly to your chest, exhaling as they go up. Lower the dumbbells slowly, taking a deep breath as they go down. Repeat.

This exercise strengthens the muscles in the upper back, the forearm and upper arm.

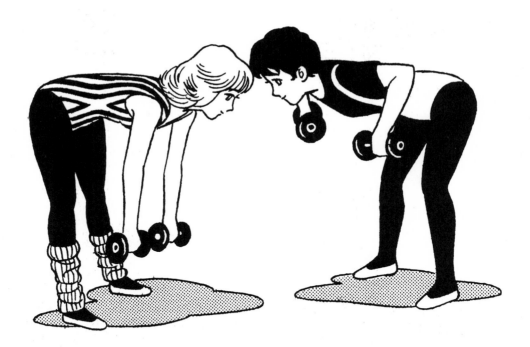

5. Deep-Knee Bends

Stand with your feet comfortably apart. If necessary, hold on to something to maintain your balance. Take a deep breath and lower your body to a squatting position. Rise back up to the starting postion, exhaling as you rise. Repeat. This exercise strengthens the thigh and hip muscles.

When you first start out, use no weights until you can easily maintain your balance while doing this exercise. When you do start using weights, this exercise may be done more comfortably with your heels raised about an inch.

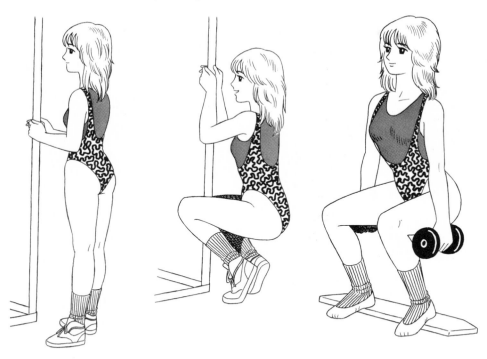

6. Shrugs

Stand with your feet about a foot apart. Hold the dumbbells hanging at your sides. Keeping your arms perfectly straight, take a deep breath and lift only your shoulders toward your ears, exhaling as you raise them. Lower your shoulders to the starting position inhaling again. Repeat.

This exercise strengthens the trapezius (the muscles from the neck to the shoulder) and neck muscles.

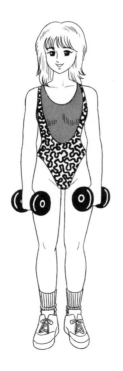 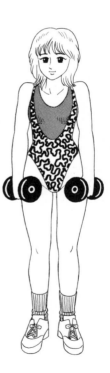

7. Head Raise

Lie on a narrow bench or across a bed with just your head hanging over the edge. Take a deep breath and raise only your head, exhaling as you raise it, keeping your shoulders flat on the bench or bed. Lower your head to the starting position while taking a deep breath.

If your neck muscles are weak, you may have trouble doing this exercise at first. You can 'cheat' a bit by not keeping your shoulders in contact with the bench. Or you can start by doing this same exercise while standing upright, then after your neck muscles strengthen, do the exercise as described above.

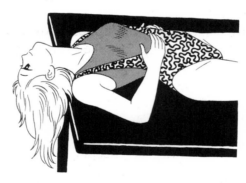

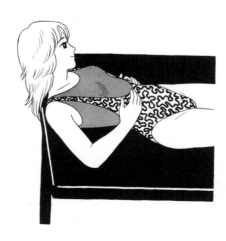

8. Situps

Lie flat on the floor and put your hands behind your head. Either have someone hold your ankles or put two or three heavy blankets over them so that your heels stay in contact with the floor. Take a deep breath and raise your upper body until your elbows touch your knees. Exhale as you come up, then take a deep breath as you lower your upper body. Repeat. Be sure to keep your legs slightly bent at the knees throughout this exercise.

This exercise strengthens the muscles in the abdomen.

If you are unable to raise your upper body until your elbows touch your knees, this exercise can be just as effective by raising your upper body only until your stomach muscles tense up, and then returning to a flat position.

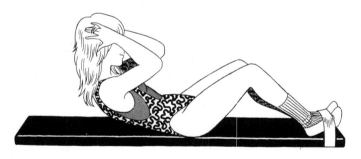

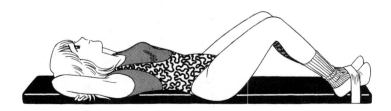

Getting Yourself in Shape

Readers of this book will probably range from those who are out of shape to those who are in good physical condition. But if you are like the average American, you are probably not in very good shape. Though some of you might be able to skip Level One below and start at Level Two, there probably aren't many who are able to complete the workout in Level Three right at the start.

Whatever level you start from, the important thing is to start slowly and be patient. Remember, it has taken a long time to gain your excess weight, so getting back to your ideal weight will also take some time. As the early chapters of this book stressed, there is no quick, magical way to lose weight without endangering your health. Although it may seem slow, the most you can expect to lose safely is about 6 pounds a month!

Level One

When you first start out, use no weights. Go through the motions of these exercises at a reasonable and deliberate pace, paying particular attention to breathing. When you are confident that you have learned how to do these exercises with the proper form, start with a light weight in each hand, and do as many repetitions as you can without strain. After you finish each exercise rest for a minute or two. A light weight is a weight that allows you to do each exercise up to about 10 or 12 repetitions.

Level Two

After a period of building up your strength and stamina your aim should be to do each of these exercises for up to about 20 repetitions, moving on to the next exercise without resting, and going through the cycle of all eight exercises. When you are in good condition, this cycle should take you about 5 minutes to complete.

Level Three

When you are able to complete Level Two comfortably, you are ready to go on to Level Three, in which you will go through the cycle more than one time, eventually without stopping. The first time you attempt Level Three, go through the whole cycle. You may be a bit winded, so rest for a couple of minutes, then proceed to go through the cycle a second time. Go as far through the cycle as you can without resting, but if you must, pause for a minute or two to catch your breath, then continue until you complete the cycle. The next workout, try to go through the cycle the second time without resting, but don't force yourself unreasonably. The important thing is that you make a bit of progress each time. When you are able to complete two cycles with a rest in between, the next step is to eliminate the rest period. In other words, go through the cycle two times without any pause. When you can do that, increase the number of times you go through the cycle to three. This should take you about 15 minutes.

Level Four (Optional)

If the workout in Level Three becomes too easy, increase the weights of the dumbells a bit. This will slow you down for a while, but when you work yourself up to the point at which you can go through three cycles of the workout with the same ease that you were able to at the lighter weight, you can be sure that your muscles have become stronger and that there has been no muscle loss because of your diet. If you want, keep increasing the weights, but don't increase them to the point at which you are unable to do at least twelve repetitions of any of the exercises. Remember, your aim is not to build big muscles, but to stimulate your muscles so they don't decrease in size.

Breathing

This type of workout is designed to increase not only your muscular strength, but also to promote pulmonary and cardiovascular fitness. In other words, it is an aerobic as well as an anaerobic workout. As such, breathing is an important part of these exercises. Be sure to breath deeply and smoothly as the instructions indicate. **Never hold your breath while performing an exercise.** One of the reasons for going through Level One without any weights is to learn how to breathe properly. By breathing deeply you emphasize the aerobic aspect of these exercises.

Recuperation

No matter what level you are at, do these workouts no more than four times a week, or every other day, yet no less than three times a week, or every third day. Whatever kind of exercise you do, your body needs to recuperate. When you exercise, you are using the energy stores in your muscles. These energy stores must be replaced and new tissue added. The body can do this only when it is at rest and getting proper nutrition. Young people recuperate relatively quickly, but as you grow older your rate of recuperation slows. It is therefore important to alternate a day of exercise with a day of no exercise. No matter how good your physical condition is, intense exercise requires recuperation.

Overtraining

When you do not allow your body time to recuperate,

symptoms of overtraining occur. Overtrained athletes become easily tired and feel sluggish most of the day, blood pressure increases, reaction time slows down, and there is a marked decrease in the ability to perform skilled movements. In effect, the body is crying out for rest.

Beginners Must Start out Slowly

Beginners of an exercise program are especially prone to this overtraining syndrome because their bodies are not used to the increased stress placed upon it. When starting on any exercise program, it is important to begin slowly, increasing the intensity gradually over a period of time.

Slow Down After Fifty

The older person who exercises should also be very cautious. The ability to endure the stress of intense exercise declines after 50 years of age even with those who have trained for most of their lives. Training for marathons or other long distance races places excessive stress on the older athlete. Cardiac arrhythmias are quite common in such persons and, although these arrhythmias in themselves may not be immediately life-threatening, any such abnormality cannot be viewed as harmless. Indeed, excessive exercise from middle age on has been proven to actually shorten life span, not lengthen it as so many promoters of the 'fitness' boom would have you believe.

Exercising When You Are Sick or Injured

When you are sick, the body needs all its strength to fight the illness, so it is not a good idea to exercise at such a time. Strenuous exercise can prolong recovery time and even increase the severity of the illness. You can console yourself during your illness with the fact that the body burns far more calories fighting a fever than it does when you are well. On a related subject, exercising too intensely before your body has adapted to the rigors of exercise can weaken your resistance. Many people start on an exercise program only to fall victim to a virus. This is another reason why you should start out very slowly.

Injuries

It is also a good idea to take a break from exercising when you are injured. This is true even when the injury isn't serious because even a minor injury can be aggravated by exercise, which could put you out of commission for a long time.

Warming Up

Warming up is an essential part of a strenuous training schedule. Unless the muscles are warm they cannot contract efficiently, so peak performance is impossible. Many injuries are caused by jumping right in and starting to train or to play some sport without properly warming up the body. Warming up does not only mean raising the heart beat and breathing hard, it also means warming up the particular muscles that will come under special strain during the course of the exercise. A baseball player should take particular care to warm up the muscles in his arms and shoulders to prepare for throwing the ball, whereas a sprinter would concentrate on thoroughly warming up the muscles in his legs and hips.

The exercises presented at the beginning of this chapter do not put excessive strain on your muscles, tendons, and joints, as long as you keep the weights used light enough so that you can do at least twelve repetitions. Still, before starting each workout it is a good idea for you to walk about briskly, and move your arms up and down over your head and swing them along your side. But avoid any jerky or abrupt motions.

Warm up the Mind as Well as the Body

Warming up also includes preparing the mind for the workout. Before exercising try to be in a relaxed state. If you are stressed out, don't exercise. Exercise is a form of stress, although a controlled kind. When you bring your outside stress with you to your workouts, control is lost.

Stretching

Stretching is an important adjunct to exercises, especially those which do not utilize the full ranges of motion of the muscles involved, such as jogging. However, stretching itself can cause injuries. When muscles are cold, they are most prone to injuries. Stretching cold muscles can cause microinjuries that become aggravated when you do the strenuous part of your training schedule. So as a basic rule you should never stretch cold muscles. Stretching is **not** warming up. You should stretch only after you have completed your exercises.

Everyone Has Different Abilities

Remember that different people have different stretching abilities. Some people have very flexible bodies with a remarkable range of movement. Others have stiffer bodies, and no matter how hard they train, they can never attain the range of motion of more flexible people. Stretching exercise can increase the range of motion of your muscles, but don't blindly follow a trainer who insists you become as flexible as rubber. The most you should do is deliberately and slowly try to reach your own limits.

When to Exercise

There is no particular time of day that you should exercise. Any time that is convenient for you is the best time. Your own unique biological rhythms may also be a factor. Some people like to exercise early in the morning, others don't. Basically, it is up to you. But it is important that you do not exercise for at least an hour after eating a meal. You also shouldn't eat for about an hour after exercising.

Exercise Will Not Take Fat off in a Specific Location

It is a waste of time to do situps or other area-specific exercises in order to take off fat only in a particular area like your stomach, waist, hips, or thighs. Certain people have a tendency to deposit fat in certain locations, women usually in the hips and thighs, men usually in the abdominal region. It is more effective to exercise the muscles throughout your whole body. In this way, you have more muscles working, which results in a higher rate of fat breakdown in your fat cells.

It is extremely difficult for women to lose fat in the hips and thighs. Lactation is the only proven way to do this. It seems that nature has reserved fat in this area primarily for the purpose of producing milk for the nourishment of a baby. Throughout pregnancy *adipose tissue lipoprotein lipase* activity in this area is extremely high, then just before the baby is born, this activity ceases and the fat is broken down and mobilized for the production of milk. Other than risking your health through very-low-calorie dieting, pregnancy is the only sure way to take off fat in this area. But since fat storage is also high during pregnancy, you will probably end up about the same amount as before.

Chapter Eight

Some Case Histories

By now you are probably wondering if this diet really works. If that's the case, you will find the following case histories fascinating. They are the stories of people who either were obese for much of their lives or became overweight because of bad personal habits.

In any event, all realized that to lead a healthier and longer life they would have to shed their extra pounds. They did it by switching to a Japanese-style diet.

Example 1

Our first case involves Roger, an American who had come to Japan at the age of 25 to study karate, but instead married a Japanese woman and settled down there.

Roger had always been physically active up until his marriage, but the responsibilities of a family forced him to work full time, leaving him little time for sports.

When he had married at 28, Roger was an athletic, lean, and fit 6 feet, 160 pounds. However, the combination of work and family pushed him into a sedentary life style. By the time he was 39, he weighed 205 pounds, had a pot belly, and could not walk up a flight of stairs without gasping for breath.

5,000 Calories a Day

The primary cause of his obesity was his Japanese wife's cooking of American-style meals. Despite being very nutritious and balanced, they were also high in fat and calories.

For example, breakfast included oatmeal or other cereals with milk, bread, cheese, eggs, and fruit. Lunches and dinners usually consisted of meat dishes with high-fat sauces and gravies, rich soups, salad with oil and vinegar as dressing, a variety of vegetables, and whole grain breads as staples. Dessert, usually consisting of cheese cake or ice cream, was seldom omitted. Roger estimated that he was gulping down 4,000 to 5,000 calories daily.

An Attack of Gout

Then, at the age of 40, Roger was struck by an attack of gout in his left foot. Blood tests showed extremely high uric acid, fat, and cholesterol levels. His doctor prescribed two medicines, one to relieve the symptoms of gout and another to lower his uric-acid levels. Additionally, the physician advised him to reduce the amount of meat he ate, to get more exercise, and to try and lose some weight.

His Exercise Program

Roger had trained actively in various sports in his youth, so he decided to start weight training and jogging. He bought a barbell with a total weight of 40 pounds and began doing various exercises. Three nights a week, promptly at six, Roger would start his training session by jogging 200 meters as a warmup, then doing a series of ten exercises with the barbell. He did this three times a week. After finishing his workout, he would take a bath and eat dinner.

Adopting the Japanese Diet

The next and critical step was a gradual switch to eating a Japanese diet. Roger began by cutting out the cheese and eggs for breakfast and all desserts. Gradually, he started to substitute fish and chicken for the meat dishes, and eliminated the high-fat gravies and sauces, using lemon, soy sauce, and other non-fat dressings instead. His daily serving of cereal and milk was eliminated and he began eating more calcium-rich dark-green vegetables plus a variety of seaweeds which guaranteed that all the essential minerals were in his diet. Within six months, Roger was eating a completely traditional Japanese diet that provided him with 2,300 calories daily.

Health and Fitness Restored

During that period he shed a total of 18 pounds. He gradually increased the intensity of his exercise, but he always kept it at a moderate level, never exercising more than 45 minutes each time nor more than three times a week. Two years after starting his regimen of diet and exercise, Roger was a trim 42-year-old man who weighed 165 pounds. He was in better physical condition than he had ever been in his life. Blood tests, taken two years after his attack of gout, showed fat and uric-acid levels had been reduced to within normal range without any medication.

Today, at 48, Roger continues following a Japanese diet combined with moderate exercise while maintaining his weight at the 160 to 165 pound level.

Roger's former life style, combining a high caloric intake and lack of exercise, was typical of many Americans. His attack of gout was an ominous warning that something was seriously wrong. Fortunately, he heeded it and today is in excellent health.

Example Two

Our next example involves an actress whose obesity was her selling point to directors needing someone to play a fat character in their movies.

At 5 feet, 6 inches, the actress weighed a staggering 215 pounds. Her diet consisted of foods high in both fat and calories. She also snacked, almost continuously, on candy, cakes, and ice cream.

However, she was depressed about her personal life and obesity, so she decided to reduce. The first thing she did was eliminate all snacks. Then she gradually reduced her caloric intake to 1,400 calories a day. Aside from that, there was nothing particularly radical about her diet. However, she ate only Japanese foods and paid particular attention to the following points:

- She used no oil in her cooking.
- She avoided all sweets and refined foods.
- She ate only fish and shellfish as the source of her animal protein.
- She ate a lot of complex carbohydrates, such as fruits, vegetables, seaweed, and brown rice, to ensure that her diet was high in fiber.
- She drank 15 glasses of water every day.
- She swam for 20 minutes every day.

Within six months she lost 45 pounds. In the next six months, she lost another 30 pounds and eventually reduced to 130 pounds. About that time, someone proposed to her and she has been happily married ever since.

Another interesting aspect of this story is that she was able to continue her work as an actress, but, needless to say, she no longer plays the role of fat women.

Example Three

This example is about another actress who also had weight problems, but the factors involved in her becoming obese were quite different than the previous example.

This actress retired from the screen after getting married. At that time she weighed only 110 pounds and was 5-feet 6-inches tall. She had three children in rapid succession, and her weight shot up to 165 pounds, the result of her voracious appetite during her pregnancies.

About six months before her first child was to enter elementary school, she decided to go on a diet because she was ashamed of her fat figure and wanted to avoid looking fat at the opening ceremony.

In a highly unusual move, she turned to boxing as her way to lose weight after the owner of a boxing gym near her home told her that boxing exercises were the best way to lose weight.

The gym owner's advice was not inaccurate. A boxer uses every muscle in his body during his training. Boxing is also aerobic. Working closely with the woman, the gym owner taught her how to shadowbox, punch a heavy bag, jump rope, and do situps. However, she did avoid getting into the ring with anyone.

She also made some minor adjustments in her diet, reducing her daily caloric intake to 1,500 calories by trimming all snacks, sweets, and foods cooked in oil, and by eating fish as her main source of animal protein.

40 Pounds of Fat Gone in Six Months

Within six months she had lost 40 pounds. Her body was as slender as it had been during her acting career, but now her muscles were firm and strong, adding an appealing vivaciousness and proportion to her body.

The above example is a case of what is referred to as *postpartum obesity*, obesity which occurs after pregnancy. This type of obesity often affects women who are restricted in their caloric intake before becoming pregnant. This example shows that it is possible for someone who has this condition to reduce through moderate caloric intake and exercises which use all the body's muscles.

Example Four

Our fourth subject involves a 5-foot 9-inch composer who shed 65 pounds in one year to achieve his ideal body weight of 180 pounds. Handicapping him was the fact that his body type was what physiologists describe as *android-type*; in simple language, his waist circumference was larger than his hip circumference. He had thick bones and large stores of fat, especially in the abdominal area. Men and women with such builds are at high risk for developing heart disease and diabetes, as well as becoming obese.

Additionally, he enjoyed a carefree life, often meeting his friends for long rounds of drinking and eating in some of Tokyo's finer Western restaurants.

Realizing that he could not continue his life style without risking his health, our subject did the following:

- He started eating only Japanese foods.
- He avoided all dishes cooked with oil.
- He reduced his intake of alcohol to one drink a day.
- He eliminated all sweets and drank his coffee black.
- He reduced his caloric intake to 1800 calories a day including the calories from his one alcoholic drink.
- He took up golf and played three times a week, allowing him to burn up calories through walking.

After following this eating pattern for about a year, he got down to about 180 pounds. At this point, he stopped losing weight, since this was the proper weight for his body type.

Example Five

Weight problems can also occur in persons who have always been healthy and lean. Sam was such a person. He never overate and he got sufficient exercise by routinely walking two miles a day to a school on the top of a hill where he taught. As a result, he was able to maintain a proper weight of 155 pounds at 5 feet 10 inches.

Then, one summer he became ill with the mumps. Initially, at the beginning of August, he didn't feel too bad, but within a few days his fever began to rise. By the middle of August his temperature reached 104 degrees, and the only thing he could do was lie in bed and hope to survive the crisis. Gradually, the fever subsided and by the end of August he had recovered.

Chicken Soup and Fruit

While he was ill he had no appetite and food tasted terrible. Chicken soup and some fruit were all he could eat.

His doctor gave him regular shots of vitamins to guard against any deficiencies. By the end of his bout with the mumps, he had lost more than 10 pounds.

An Uncontrollable Appetite

Then on the morning of the last day of August, he awoke with a ravenous appetite. He ate two eggs scrambled in butter with ham, three pieces of toast, a bowl of cereal with milk, and some fruit. Surprisingly, for a man who had never overeaten, it was not enough. He asked his wife to prepare more ham and eggs with toast. Still, the additional serving did not satisfy him and he nibbled on bits of food all morning. That day, he ate a huge lunch followed by an enormous dinner.

For the next three months he continued these eating patterns until one day a friend remarked how much weight he had gained. He looked down and discovered that his now bulging belly nearly prevented him from seeing his feet. When he weighed himself later, the scales stopped at 174 pounds. He had gained a hefty 19 pounds since his illness.

A Happy Ending

This story had a happy ending. Sam cut down on his abnormally high intake of food and started to do some jogging in addition to his regular hill climbing. But this example clearly shows that severe food restriction, even in a person without a previous weight problem, can initiate metabolic changes which produce intense cravings for food and a propensity for the body to store fat.

While this was a highly unusual case, I have presented it to show that anyone can face a weight problem which, if left uncorrected, could ruin your health.

Chapter Nine

The Five Basic Principles for Losing Weight

There is no doubt that obesity is caused by the high-fat, high-calorie diets of modern, affluent societies. Of all the rich nations of the world, Japan is the only one where obesity is still only a minor problem. Overweight or obese people do, of course, exist in this country. Japan has a diverse culture in which many different life styles are represented. But the problem is kept in check by the traditional Japanese diet, to which most of the people on these islands adhere with an almost religious zeal.

The Diet Most Suited to Our Digestive Metabolisms

Of all the diets in the world today, the traditional Japanese diet corresponds most closely to the diet our digestive metabolisms are suited to accommodate. It is a diet low in fat, high in protein, and high in complex carbohydrates. Were the people in Western countries to adopt the Japanese-style diet presented in this book or in my previous book, *East Meets West, Supernutrition from Japan*, their incidence of obesity, heart disease, cancer, and other 'adult diseases' would be drastically lowered.

A Diet for Health and Longevity

Even if you do not eat a Japanese diet, there are a number of principles which this diet can teach you. If you follow them in the choice of your foods, you can expect greater health, longevity, and a lean and fit body for the rest of your life. The advantage of incorporating the Japanese diet as it is presented here into your daily meals is that it has already been planned for you, so you don't have to study nutrition in order to develop your menus.

The Five Basic Principles

There are countless things that people tell you *not* to do. Don't smoke, don't drink, don't eat sweets, etc. Of all these things smoking is clearly the most damaging to the body, but most 'recreational' foods won't hurt you if they are eaten in moderation. They may even be beneficial in that they help relieve stress. Even an occasional feast or 'pig out' won't hurt you if you are in good health. The important thing, however, is to establish a pattern of eating and life style that incorporate the following five principles:

- **Caloric intake must approximately equal energy expenditure.** Depending on body size, sex, and level of activity this can, on average, range from 1,400 calories to 2,500 calories a day.

- **Fat intake is necessary, but must be kept low (around 20% of total calories).** Moreover, there must be a balance between the different kinds of fats, with fats from fish and plant sources represented, while saturated fats from beef should be kept at a minimum.

- **Complex carbohydrates must constitute about 60% of total daily calories.** They provide the body with its basic energy needs. Complex carbohydrates are fruits, vegetables, grains, potatoes, nuts, and beans.

- **Protein is an important nutrient that must be present in the daily diet in adequate amounts.** The real danger of eating meat is not that you will get too much protein, but that you will get too much fat. On the other hand, excessive protein intake is not good either. But if caloric intake is kept moderate and the percentage of the complex carbohydrate intake is kept above 60% of total calories, it is impossible to eat too much protein.

- **An active body is essential for maintaining ideal weight and health.** If you cannot expend sufficient energy through your daily activities, you must exercise. Without muscular movement, the body loses its metabolic efficiency, and obesity is the inevitable result. But like overeating, overexercising can also harm the body. In all things, moderation is the key.

Almost anyone can become more active with a little effort. The difficult thing is eating properly, because it requires knowledge of the kinds of foods you should eat. But by adding the traditional Japanese meals described in the following pages, you will automatically be adhering to the first four principles, giving you the foundation for fitness, health, and longevity.

Remember, you diet not to lose weight, but to ensure that you live a long life in good health. A slim, fit, and beautiful body is simply the natural result of this.

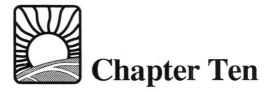 **Chapter Ten**

Implementing the Program

Changing Your Life Style

If you want to lose your excess weight and keep it off, you will have to make permanent changes in your diet. Specifically, you must incorporate the Japanese principles of eating and avoid a sedentary life style. The program presented in these pages, including the exercise routines and the menus and recipes in the next chapters, can be used as a model for your new pattern of diet and exercise. In short, it is a beginner's course to teach you the principles of correct living.

It is not necessary to follow the exercise program exactly as described. There are a lot of other beneficial ways to exercise. In fact, if you are active and move around a lot in your daily activities, using all the muscles in your body, it may not be necessary for you to exercise at all. Actually, this is the way nature intended you to exercise. But the sedentary life styles of modern societies force us to invent artificial means to give our bodies the activity they require.

Primitive Man Did a Lot of Walking

Before the advent of modern society, human beings did a

lot of brisk walking searching for food. It is estimated that early men and women covered at least 2 to 3 miles a day. And their activity wasn't limited to walking. They also ran a lot, lifted and carried heavy things and climbed trees. So early man used all of his muscles, and his daily activities were both aerobic and anaerobic.

There are many things you can do to increase your level of activity. If you take a bus or train to work, get up a bit earlier and briskly walk one or two stations before boarding your bus or train. If you work in an office building, don't take the elevator to your office, climb the stairs instead. Some of these suggestions may not be practical for your particular life style, but if you think about it, you can find ways to increase the amount of activity you do every day.

A Diet That Can Make You Lose Weight

The menus presented in the next chapter are examples of low-fat yet highly nutritious meals that can help you lose weight. You can plan your own menus and recipes based on these examples, remembering that emphasis on Japanese foods and fish is by far the simplest way to make sure that your diet is low in fat, low in calories, yet nutritionally balanced.

Start Out Slowly

A major flaw in almost all other diet programs is that they start you out on a "crash" program. They urge you to drop your food intake from a half to a third of what you are used to. This is a great shock to the body, which interprets this drop in calories as a time of famine and starts to build up high levels of *adipose tissue lipoprotein lipase*, the enzyme discussed in Chapters Two and Six that plays an important role in the storage of fat.

Exercising is the Same

Exercising involves a similar kind of change. If you are living a sedentary life, you cannot suddenly jump into a strenuous, intensive exercise program until you have built up the strength, stamina, and cardiovascular and pulmonary fitness to withstand the stress that such a program imposes on the body. In both dieting and exercise, you must start out slowly in order to gradually accustom your body to the changes necessary to lose weight.

A Preparation Period

Before you start out on this program you will have to make some preparations. You will have to find out where to buy many of the ingredients necessary for preparing the recipes described here. You will have to learn how to cook Japanese style. But you can use this preparation period as a time to accustom your body to the changes in store for it. The whole process will take time. You cannot get a new and beautiful body both instantly and safely.

Analyzing Your Present Diet

Look at your present diet. What are some of the things in it that are unnecessary? Make a list of all the things you eat in a week. Which are high-fat or high-calorie foods? The first thing you can do is cut out desserts. Instead of a sugary snack, eat fresh fruit. Remember, sweets contain seven times more calories per ounce than fruit, and they are usually loaded with fat. By eating fresh fruit for dessert you can eliminate at least 300 to 400 calories per day.

In preparation for regularly eating Japanese food, you might start substituting rice for bread and fish for beef with some of your meals. With judicious pruning, you could gradually eliminate from 500 to 1,000 calories a day. After a couple of weeks, you could be at the 2,500 calorie level.

How Many Calories a Day is Right for You?

The most important question you have to answer for yourself is 'How many calories a day are right for me?' Nutritionists often say that 2,000 calories a day are necessary for maintainance. As an average, this may be correct, but clearly a person with a large build needs more calories for maintainance than a small person.

Women, being on average smaller than men, generally eat less. Not only are women smaller, but they have, on average, a higher percentage of body fat and a lower percentage of muscle than a man. Fat is nearly metabolically inert, while muscle is metabolically quite active, even when at rest. Therefore, fat contributes almost nothing to *basal metabolism*. This means that a woman's basal metabolic rate is lower than a man's, so she requires less energy intake than a man of the same size.

If you make further reductions in your caloric intake once you have reached your ideal weight, the body will resist additional weight loss by lowering its basal metabolic rate. But there is a limit to how far this can be lowered. To understand this it is necessary to define basal metabolism.

Basal Metabolism

The cells in the body must be continually active in order to maintain life processes. The internal organs, such as the liver and kidneys, are constantly functioning. The heart is beating and the lungs are breathing, while the muscles cause your chest to expand and contract. The brain is also actively consuming energy, using as much as 20% of the energy the body expends at rest. Even when sleeping, the muscles maintain their tone, using about 25% of the resting energy of your body. These basic physiological processes are known as *basal metabolism*.

Basal Metabolic Rate

Physiologists often speak of *basal metabolic rate* (BMR). This is the amount of energy used during a fixed period of time when you are lying quietly but awake, at a comfortable temperature, 12 to 15 hours after eating. BMR varies from person to person. It depends on age, sex, and body size. It can also be affected by certain endocrine disorders. Even eatinglarge amounts or small amounts of food can change it. BMR is very high in infants and children, but gradually decreases through adolescence. In adulthood it gradually declines at a very slow rate with advancing age.

BMR Varies with Weight

BMR varies relative to weight and height, but from just your weight, you can roughly determine the amount of energy your basal metabolism consumes during a 24-hour period using one of two formulas, one for men and the other for women.

For men the formula is:

11 calories times body weight in pounds =
energy consumed in a 24-hour period by basal metabolism.

For women, it is slightly lower:

10 calories times body weight in pounds =
energy consumed in a 24-hour period by basal metabolism.

Using these formulas a 160-pound man would use

11 x 160 = 1,760 calories in 24 hours.

A 110-pound women would use

10 x 110 = 1,100 calories in 24 hours.

These formulas are generally applicable for adults in their 20's. As a person grows older his BMR gradually decreases.

Daily Activities Burn Additional Calories

Bear in mind that BMR is just the energy your body needs to keep functioning at a minimum level. You are going to have to use additional calories when you move around, work, exercise, etc. You even need extra calories to digest your food. Therefore, to calculate the daily calories your body needs you must also take these factors into consideration.

To illustrate, a 110-pound woman doing light housework would need to add about 600 calories over her BMR to calculate how many calories she is using each day. A 160-pound man or women sitting all day at a desk in an office may need to add the same amount over his or her BMR to get an idea of the number of calories burned each day.

Getting on the 'Razor's Edge'

As previously mentioned, when the number of calories eaten falls below the number of calories your body needs to maintain itself, the body can compensate by lowering its BMR. But there is a limit to how low basal metabolic rate can be. The trick to losing fat is to try to get on that 'razor's edge' where the calories eaten are just about the same as the calories burned up by activity. At that point, if you are stimulating your muscles to grow, the body will have to use your fat stores to get the energy it needs. This is how you can 'turn' fat into muscle.

Reduce Caloric Intake Gradually

By using this method of gradually dropping calories, you will be able to determine your own individual 'razor's edge'. When you start losing weight you will be burning up more calories than you are consuming. But this caloric deficit will be slight and, as long as it is not carried on for too long, it will not harm you. There will come a time, however, when you will stop losing weight. At this point, slightly increase the number of calories eaten. If you continue with the exercise program, you should be able to maintain your newly-achieved weight. Just remember one thing. Dropping the number of calories you eat every day below your BMR can be *very* dangerous. As I've repeatedly mentioned, when this happens, muscle tissue is torn down and *adipose tissue lipoprotein lipase* starts to increase until you resume your normal eating patterns. When normal eating does resume, this enzyme goes into action, causing a high rate of fat storage.

No Magic Number

As you can see there is no magic number of calories that you must eat everyday. Everyone is different. You have to determine for yourself at what level of caloric intake you will start to lose weight. Short of living in the metabolic ward of a hospital, where your food intake is measured to the milligram and your caloric expenditure is constantly monitored, the only way you can do this is by gradually reducing your caloric intake until you start losing weight.

Step by Step

In summary, the first stage of this diet and exercise program is the preparatory stage during which you start reducing the amount of fat, refined foods, sugar, and the number of calories you eat each day. In the second stage, you eat about 2,500 calories a day, including a lot of Japanese food. At this point you should be at Level Two in the exercise program. If you start losing weight, continue at the 2,500 calorie level. If not, after about two to three weeks, go down to about 2,200 calories, continuing with the exercise program while gradually increasing its intensity. If you are still not losing weight, go down to 1,900 calories. Continue the downward progression of calories with increased intensity in the exercise program until you are losing weight. At some point, you will reach that 'razor's edge' where you will be taking off fat and maintaining muscle size. You will also be eating an ideal diet, a diet that will lower your risk for heart disease and cancer and enable you to live a long, healthy and vigorous life.

Chapter Eleven

How to Start Losing Weight by Eating Japanese Foods

Now that you have learned the problems with eating Western-style foods and how Japanese-style foods can solve some of those problems, you are ready to begin losing weight. Just apply the five basic principles to your own diet.

Gradually Reduce Your Caloric Intake

Begin gradually reducing your food consumption to the 2,500-calorie-a-day level. If you are a typical American, you are currently eating 3,000 to 4,000 calories a day, so reducing your food intake to 2,500 calories a day should be done over a few weeks. If you have a large frame and you exercise, you may find that you will lose weight at the 2,500-calorie level, but most people have to get below the 2,000-calorie-a-day level before they notice significant results. Gradually decrease your caloric intake until you have reached a level at which you are losing weight. *I cannot emphasize enough that you must reduce your caloric intake gradually so that you do not give your body a sudden shock.*

Listen to Your Body

It is also important to listen to what your body tells you. Lack of energy plus weight loss can mean that you are below the minimum daily required calories. If this is the case, slightly raise your caloric intake to the point where your energy is restored but you are still losing weight. In any event, do not eat less than 1,400 calories without the advice of your doctor. An exception to this would be if you are well below average height and build so that your body does not require so many calories. *Remember that very-low-calorie diets are dangerous. Don't take chances.*

As you begin your new exercise and eating habits, always keep in mind that the selection of the right foods in your diet is of the utmost importance. If you only reduce calories by eating the same kinds of high-fat foods, you will become frustrated and hungry without achieving your goals. Substituting low-fat, high-carbohydrate Japanese meals for Western ones will allow you to reduce your calorie count without hunger and, just as importantly, without skimping on your nutritional requirements.

Cut Down on Fat

Cut down on your consumption of fats, especially saturated fats. You can make significant progress by eating more fish and chicken (without skin) and eating beef and pork only occasionally. Your goal should be to make fat account for no more than 20% of your total calories. Remember, however, *vegetable oils are essential to your health,* and they are used in many of the recipes in Chapter Fourteen. The important thing is not to overuse them and to choose the right kinds. Most oils commercially sold in Japan are a blend of rapeseed (*natane*) and soybean oil, and this results in a healthy fatty-acid profile (rapeseed oil in particular has an ideal fatty-acid profile). Unlike most other oils, both are high in an omega-3 fatty acid (alpha-linolenic acid) which has beneficial effects on health. Olive oil is another vegetable oil that I recommend using. It is high in a monounsaturated fatty acid (oleic acid) which has also been shown to give protection against heart disease. Most other vegetable oils, such as safflower oil, are too high in a polyunsaturated fatty acid (linoleic acid), and you should be careful about consuming too much of them.

Eat More Complex Carbohydrates

Avoid the empty calories of sugary snacks. Increase the amount of complex carbohydrates you eat by choosing brown rice and whole-grain breads. Sweet potatoes, with their high level of nutrients, make a healthy snack. Eliminate sugary desserts and dairy foods that have a high-fat content. Cakes, cookies, pastries, and candy not only have enormous amounts of sugar, but usually have a high percentage of fat. Fatty dairy products, such as sour cream, whipped cream, ice cream, and butter should also be strictly limited. If you must have desserts, switch to fresh fruit.

Losing Weight Is a Long-Term Project

Adopting this way of eating is a long-term project. You have spent many years becoming overweight. There is no safe way that you can get back to your ideal weight in a short period of time.

The remainder of this chapter contains fourteen tasty and nutritious Japanese meals. Substitute these in place of your Western-style dinners or lunches. You need not eat Japanese food exclusively, but the more often you eat in the Japanese way, the easier you will find it to reduce the amount of calories and fat you eat.

These meals are made up of typical dishes served in Japanese homes. Many follow the traditional meal structure described in Chapter Four. The casserole, or 'one-pot meal' is also represented. Because these meals include only fish, shellfish, and chicken without skin, they are low in saturated fats. Protein intake is high but not excessive, while fat intake is low but adequate. Complex carbohydrates make up the balance and the bulk of these meals, supplying the starch you need for energy. Their high fiber content will also help eliminate toxic wastes from your body and maintain optimal blood levels of fat, sugar, and insulin.

You will find recipes for each of the dishes in these meals in Chapter Thirteen. These are identical to the meals people eat in Japan except that I have reduced the use of sugar and salt. If you are attempting to restrict your consumption of salt, you may want to cut back on the amount of soy sauce used in some of these recipes.

I have not included traditional Japanese breakfast menus because it is a bit unreasonable to expect Americans to eat a 100% Japanese diet. Nowadays, even Japanese don't do this. Breakfast, however, is important. It should supply about a third of your calories. Neglecting to eat breakfast is the worst thing you can do when you are trying to lose weight. When you get up in the morning you usually haven't eaten for 12 hours. If you go through the whole morning without eating, the body interprets this as a time of famine and gears itself up to store fat.

Oatmeal Is the Ideal Breakfast Food

However, don't eat a breakfast high in sugars and fat. Start the day, instead, by carefully selecting Western foods that will help you achieve that slim and healthy figure you desire. Oatmeal, with its high-pectin content, is an excellent food for people who want to lose weight. I strongly urge you to eat it for breakfast often, mixed with fresh fruit and low-fat milk. Whole-grain bread can be substituted for oatmeal. However, avoid high-calorie butter or jams. Try the fresh soybean jam, the recipe for which is shown on page 146. Eating a soft boiled egg with your toast is also a fine combination. Eggs are a highly nutritious food and there is nothing wrong with eating them two or three times a week.

In the meals below fat averages less than 18% of calories, yet there is enough to satisfy your minimum requirements. Protein averages about 24% per meal. This may seem high, but remember that a healthy breakfast of fruit, bread or other grains will be high in carbohydrates, so the percentage of protein intake per day with respect to total daily calories should be below 20%. Moreover, a high-carbohydrate afternoon snack of fruit, which has almost no protein or fat, will also bring your percentage of protein and fat intake even lower. Another point to bear in mind is that these meals average less than 500 calories a day. This is rather low and will not be enough for many people, so you should increase the amount of rice from one cup to as much as needed to bring your energy intake up to the level of your energy expenditure. This will also lower the ratio of your protein intake. Remember, everybody has different calorie requirements and it is impossible to set a standard that will hold for everyone. You must determine for yourself based on the information given in this book what your own requirements are.

Fourteen Japanese Meals for Losing Weight

Most of these meals come with a serving of rice. This is assumed to be one cup of cooked rice and consists of 4% fat, 7% protein, and 89% carbohydrates.

The recipes are given in Chapter Thirteen.

Meal One
Wakame Soup: 61 calories
Boiled Chicken Mixed with Vegetables: 102 calories
Tofu with Daikon Leaves: 119 calories
Rice: 230 calories
492 calories; 18% fat; 25% protein; 57% carbohydrate; 1.4g sodium

Meal Two
Sole Stew: 70 calories
Boiled Hijiki, Carrots and Deep-Fried Tofu Puffs: 96 calories
Rice: 230 calories
396 calories; 15% fat; 23% protein; 62% carbohydrates; 0.3g sodium

Meal Three
Pumpkin and Shiitake Miso Soup: 70 calories
Chicken and Cashew Nuts: 145 calories
Cauliflower Salad: 87 calories
Rice: 230 calories
532 calories; 25% fat; 28% protein; 47% carbohydrates; 0.7g sodium

Meal Four
Wakame and Tofu Miso Soup: 64 calories
Mackerel with Tomato and Onion Dressing: 185 calories
Tofu and Vegetable Mix: 90 calories
Rice: 230 calories
569 calories; 29% fat; 20% protein; 51% carbohydrates; 1.2g sodium

Meal Five

Egg and Leek Soup: 65 calories
Steamed Chicken: 117 calories
Boiled Komatsuna: 37 calories
Rice: 230 calories
449 calories; 12% fat; 31% protein; 57% carbohydrates; 0.9g sodium

Meal Six

Brocolli and Tofu Soup: 43 calories
Sardines in Umeboshi Sauce: 93 calories
Brussel Sprouts and Carrot Salad with Egg-Strip Topping: 103 calories
Rice: 230 calories
469 calories; 20% fat; 16% protein; 62% carbohydrates; 1.8g sodium

Meal Seven

Clam Miso Soup: 36 calories
Chicken and Eggs on Rice: 292 calories
Vinegared Daikon and Carrots: 120 calories
448 calories; 18% fat; 28% protein; 54% carbohydrates; 1.3g sodium

Meal Eight

Kamaboko and Snow-Pea Soup: 30 calories
Shrimp, Squid, and Brocolli: 190 calories
Carrot Salad: 91 calories
Rice: 230 calories
550 calories; 20% fat; 20% protein; 60% carbohydrates; 0.9g sodium

Meal Nine

Clam Soup: 31 calories
Boiled Chicken and Sweet Potatoes: 208 calories
Daikon, Carrots, and Cucumber Salad: 47 calories
Rice: 230 calories
516 calories; 13% fat; 25% protein; 62% carbohydrates; 1.1g sodium

Meal Ten
Potato and Green-Onion Miso Soup: 86 calories
Salmon Saute 167 calories
Boiled Komatsuna and Bean Sprouts: 21 calories
Rice: 230 calories
504 calories; 18% fat; 25% protein; 57% carbohydrates; 0.7g sodium

Meal Eleven
Komatsuna and Deep-Fried Tofu Puffs Miso Soup: 125 calories
Chicken and Chinese Cabbage: 131 calories
Okara: 70 calories
Rice: 230 calories
556 calories; 18% fat; 26% protein; 56% carbohydrates; 1.7g sodium

Meal Twelve
Boiled Yellowtail: 300 calories
Hijiki and Sesame Seeds: 90 calories
Rice: 160 calories
484 calories; 18% fat; 19% protein; 63% carbohydrates; 1.3g sodium

Meal Thirteen
Chicken Casserole: 144 calories
Rice: 230 calories
374 calories; 10% fat; 30% protein; 60% carbohydrates; 0.1g sodium

Meal Fourteen
Fish Casserole: 494 calories
Udon: 45 calories
539 calories; 9% fat; 27% protein; 66% carbohydrates; 1.8g sodium

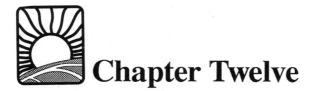

Chapter Twelve

How to Make Soups, Rice and Vegetables

Soups and Stock

One of the most important elements in Japanese cooking is the soup stock, or *dashi* as the Japanese call it. Not only is it essential to the preparation of soup, but it also plays a role in the cooking of many of the other dishes served.

The common ingredient in all Japanese stock is the seaweed kombu (kelp). You can either make stock with kelp alone, or with dried bonito flakes or dried sardines.

Most Japanese housewives use packaged stock in powdered form, a time-saving convenience. While the taste of the better products is excellent, you may want to make the stock yourself to ensure that you get all the nutrients you can from the kelp and other ingredients.

Making Stock with Kelp

Use a 6-inch strip of dried kelp. When you first take it out the package it will be covered with a white substance. Wipe it off with a damp cloth. Soak the kelp in 4 cups of water for about an hour, then heat the water. Just as the water begins to boil, remove the kelp from the water.

Stock with Kelp and Bonito Flakes or Dried Sardines

Basic Stock (used for clear soups)
Follow the procedure above for making stock with kelp, then add 1/4 of a cup of water and heat. Just as the stock is about to boil, add 1 cup of bonito flakes. As it is boiling, foam will begin to rise. At this point lower the flame and let it simmer for 10 seconds. Turn off the flame and add a pinch of salt. The bonito flakes will sink to the bottom. Immediately strain; it is now ready for use.

Secondary Stock (used for thick soups and cooking oden)
In this stock you use the kelp and bonito flakes left over from making basic stock. Add 4 cups of water and heat. When it starts to boil, lower the flame and let it simmer for 15 minutes. Immediately strain and store for use.

Stock with Dried Sardines (usually used for miso soups)
Wash and then soak about 10 small dried sardines in 5 cups of water for up to 3 hours (the longer you soak them, the stronger the stock). Heat to about 100 degrees fahrenheit and strain.

Miso Soups and Clear Soups

In the traditional Japanese diet there are two main kinds of soups served: miso soups (*misoshiru*) and clear soups (*suimono*). These soups can be made in a number of variations by altering the ingredients used, but the base of these two types of soups remains the same. Miso soups are made using a soup stock and miso. Clear soups are made using only basic stock.

Different kinds of soups can be made by adding two or more types of vegetables, or a vegetable and fish or tofu. here are some examples of miso and clear soups.

Clear Soups

Chicken and Shimeji Soup
(serves four)

Ingredients

30 grams white chicken meat

1/2 pack of shimeji

4 cups of soup stock

1/2T of soy sauce

1/2t salt

Directions

Boil the chicken for about 3 minutes. Shred into small pieces. Cut the shimeji into bite size pieces and boil for one minute.

Divide the chicken and shimeji into four soup bowls. Pour the stock over it and serve.

34 calories; 9% fat; 79% protein; 39% carbohydrates; 0.4g sodium (per serving)

Red Snapper Soup
(serves four)

Ingredients

6 oz. red snapper or any other white fish

3 scallions, chopped

3 cups stock

1/2t of salt

1/2t of sake

1t of soy sauce

yuzu (citron) or lemon peels

Directions

Salt fish and let stand for 10 minutes. Heat stock, add soy sauce and sake, and bring to a boil. Add fish and boil until cooked. To serve, put on portion of fish into a soup bowl, add stock and garnish with scallions and citrus peels.

51 calories; 6% fat; 64% protein; 10% carbohydrates; 0.1g sodium (per serving)

Miso Soups

Potato and Wakame Miso soup
(serves four)

Ingredients

1 potatoes   5T of miso paste
2 oz wakame   4 cups of stock

Directions

Boil potatoes in stock until tender. Add wakame to boiling stock. Dissolve miso in some boiling stock. Stir into soup. Heat and serve.

80 calories; 14% fat; 40% protein; 45% carbohydrates; 1.1g sodium (per serving)

Other Combinations

Once you have learned to make Japanese soups with the examples given above, you can experiment with other variations. Here are a few combinations that you can use for soups, both miso and clear soups.

- Bamboo shoots and wakame
- Clams and shiitake
- Chicken with a vegetable or seaweed
- White fish and scallions

Rice Dishes

How to Cook Rice

Measure out the amount of rice you will need and put it a bowl of water. Rinse and drain a number of times until the water is clear. Soak for about 30 minutes to one hour to allow the rice to absorb water.

Put the rice in a cooking pot with slightly more water than rice and leave it on a medium flame until the water boils. After it begins to boil, increase to a high flame for about one minute. Next boil it over a low flame for up to 5 minutes. At this point reduce the flame to as low as possible, and boil this way for 10 minutes. Turn off the flame and let stand for 10 minutes. The rice is now ready.

Nowadays, almost all families in Japan use automatic rice cookers to prepare rice. Using this appliance ensures getting perfectly cooked rice every time. The thermostat controls increase and decrease the heat in the cooker at exactly the right time. There are also markers inside, indicating the exact proportion of rice to water to use. These rice cookers are available at many oriental food stores. When cooking brown rice, it is best to use a pressure cooker.

Rice is usually served by itself in a bowl. However, it is eaten with the other dishes, so the flavors of the other foods enhance the bland taste of the rice. For breakfast, Japanese will often mix small dried fish, bonito flakes, or *natto* with their rice. Rice served with a meal may even be mixed with vegetables or other ingredients. However, Japanese eat many concoctions in which rice is the central ingredient. Three important kinds of such rice dishes are rice porridges (*zosui*), rice with bamboo shoots (*takenoko gohan*), and rice gruel (okayu), a kind of overboiled rice.

Rice and Crab Vegetable Porridge
(serves four)

This is a breakfast dish often served to those who are ill or have a hangover. The ingredients can be changed to suit your taste.

Ingredients

3 cups of rice
4 cups of soup stock
1 cake of soft tofu
4 oz. grams of crab sticks

1 bunch of trefoil (mitsuba)
2 scrambled eggs
a dash of salt
2t of sake

Directions

Cut the tofu into bite-size pieces, the crab sticks and the trefoil (mitsuba) into 1-inch lengths. Put the rice and soup stock in a covered earthenware casserole with a high flame. As soon as it comes to a boil, remove the cover, reduce to a low flame, and add the tofu and crab sticks. Return to a boil, add the sake and salt, and stir. Next pour in the scrambled eggs while stirring, add the trefoil, and turn off the flame. Put on the lid and steam until the eggs are soft boiled.

250 calories; 9% fat; 25% protein; 66% carbohydrates; 0.1g sodium (per serving)

Rice and Bamboo Shoots (serves four)

Ingredients

3 cups rice
1/3 lb boiled bamboo shoots
1/2 cup sake
1T light soy sauce

2t of mirin (sweet sake)
1/2t salt
an appropriate quantity of
trefoil (mitsuba) stems

Directions

Thoroughly wash rice and let stand for about 30 minutes. Cut the bamboo shoots into thin bite-sized pieces and soak together with a mixture of the mirin light soy sauce, sake, and salt. Briefly boil the trefoil stems. In a casserole, place the rice with 3-1/3 cups of water plus the bamboo mixture and stir. When the bamboo shoots rise to the surface, boil briefly, remove from heat and serve. When serving, sprinkle the trefoil stems on the top.

226 calories; 3% fat; 9% protein; 88% carbohydrates; 0.5g sodium (per serving)

Rice Gruel with Umeboshi (serves four)

This is the traditional Japanese dish served to people who are ill with a cold the flu. It has the same mystique as chicken soup has in the United States.

Ingredients

  4 cups of rice   4 umeboshis (pickled plums)

Directions

    In a pan or casserole, pour 4 cups of rice that has already been cook and bring to a boil over a high flame with the cover on the pot. When it starts to boil, remove the lid and simmer over a low flame. Don't mix too much, but on the other hand do not allow the rice to stick to the casserole and burn.

    When the rice gets soft and expands, it is ready to serve. Put in a bowl with an umeboshi on top with each serving. As an option, you can add and mix in small pieces of meat or fish, or other condiments to your taste.

235 calories; 4% fat; 7% protein; 89% carbohydrates; 0.8g sodium (per serving)

Salmon Ochazuke
(serves four)

    Ochazuke is a tasty and nutritious rice-soup concoction. It makes an especially satisfying dish in the cold winter months as a light meal when a bland bowl of rice may not quite hit the spot. The main ingredients are rice and nori with a dab of wasabi added. In place of salmon, pollock roe or umeboshi are commonly used.

Ingredients

4 oz. baked salmon	a dash of salt
4 cups of rice that has been cooked	4T of sake
4 cups of soup stock	4 sheets nori cut into strips

Directions

    Remove the skin and bones from the salmon and tear into small (1/2-inch square) chunks. Add the salt and sake to the stock and bring to a boil. Put the rice in a bowl and lay the cut nori over it. Sprinkle with some sesame seed if you choose and put the salmon on top. Finally, add a bit (1/4-inch cube) of wasabi and pour the hot soup stock into the bowl. Serve with a lid covering the bowl.

293 calories; 7% fat; 16% protein; 77% carbohydrates; 0.1g sodium (per serving)

Rice and Barley (Mugimeshi)

Japanese usually eat white rice, and many of the nutrients are lost in the polishing process. To make up for this loss, it is a common practice for Japanese to add barley to their rice. The usual rice and barley mixture is 70% rice to 30% barley, depending on an individual's taste.

Directions

Wash the rice and barley in water several times, and soak for 30 minutes. To each cup of rice and barley add an equal amount of water and cook the same way you would ordinary rice.

Rice Balls

Rice balls are made with a ball of rice, usually with salmon, umeboshi, or cod roe inserted inside, and wrapped with a sheet of nori. They are a nice variation to ordinary rice and are delicious, nutritious, and filling afternoon snacks. If you make these rice balls by hand, keep 1/2 cup of salted water handy to dip your fingers into so that the rice doesn't stick to your fingers. Alternatively, you can use a wooden triangular mold to make rice balls. In this case, you fill up the mold with rice, putting whatever filling you desire in the middle, put the top on and press.

The recipes below serve eight persons.

Tarako Rice Balls

Ingredients

five cups of rice

2 tarako

1/2 cup of salted water (1/2t salt)

Direction

Bake the roe with the outer skin still intact for about 10 minutes wrapped in aluminium foil. When done shred the roe and spread on the outside of the rice ball as shown in the photo.

158 calories; 4% fat; 15% protein; 81% carbohydrates; 0.7g sodium (per serving)

Umeboshi Rice Balls

Ingredients
5 cups of rice
4 umeboshi
3 sheets of yakinori

1/2 cup of salted water (1/2t of salt)

Direction
Take the seeds out of the umeboshi and shred into eight to ten pieces. Mold the rice into balls and put some umeboshi in each and cover with nori as shown in the photo.

146 calories; 4% fat; 8% protein; 88% carbohydrates; 0.8g sodium (per serving)

Salmon Rice Balls

Ingredients
5 cups of rice
baked salmon
1/2 sheet nori slightly singed

1/2 cup of salted water (1/2t of salt)

Directions
Shred the salmon into pieces and mix together with the rice. Make into rice balls and wrap with nori as shown in the photo.

163 calories; 6% fat; 14% protein; 80% carbohydrates; 0.1g sodium (per serving)

Parsley Rice Balls

Ingredients
5 cups of rice
2T of chopped parsley
some bonito flakes

1/2t of salt
1/2 cup of salted water (1/2t of salt)

Direction
Mix the parsley, rice, and salt together and make into rice balls. Add bonito flakes if desired.

144 calories; 4% fat; 7% protein; 89% carbohydrates; 0.3g sodium (per serving)

Mixed Vegetables Rice Balls

Ingredients

5 cups of rice

1/4 cup of frozen mixed vegetables

1/2 cup of salted water (1/2t of salt)

Direction

Boil the vegetables until done. Mix together with rice and salt.

146 calories; 4% fat; 7% protein; 89% carbohydrates; 0.1g sodium (per serving)

Boiled Green Vegetables

The Japanese boil their vegetables for a brief period so that few nutrients are lost in the boiling process. After they are cooked, the vegetable is rinsed in cold water. The excess water is then either squeezed, drained or shaken off. This way of cooking vegetables is called *ohitashi* in Japanese. The dish below is a typical example.

Shungiku and Sesame Seeds (serves four)

Ingredients

2 bunches shungiku (a green herb called chrysanthemum leaves)

3T white sesame seeds

a dash of sugar

a dash of soy sauce

a dash of sake

Directions

Boil shungiku until it darkens. Rinse with cold water, cut into 1-inch lengths and squeeze the water out with your hands.

Stir fry sesame seeds, sake and soy sauce in a frying pan. Mix the shungiku with the sugar in a bowl and sprinkle the sesame seeds.

39 calories; 63% fat; 23% protein; 14% carbohydrates; 0.1g sodium (per serving)

The Japanese Alternative for Weight Loss

 Ingredients

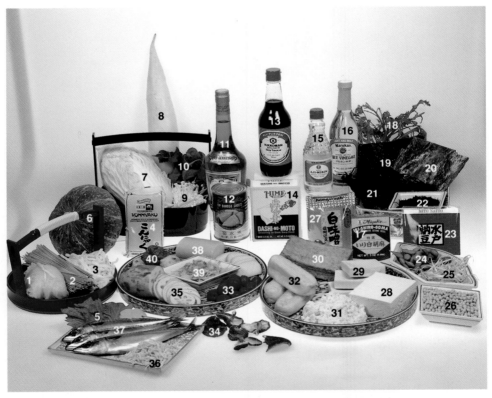

1. shirataki	13. soy sauce	27. miso
2. soba	14. dashi no moto	28. tofu
3. udon	15. mirin	29. koya-dofu
4. konnyaku	16. rice vinegar	30. atsuage
5. shiso	17. sesame seeds	31. okara
6. japanese pumpkin	18. shungiku	32. aburage
(kabocha)	19. nori	33. umeboshi
7. hakusai	20. konbu	34. shiitake
8. daikon	21. wakame	35. lotus root
9. enokitake mushrooms	22. hijiki	36. shirasuboshi
10. trefoil (mitsuba)	23. natto	37. saba
11. sake	24. edamame	38. kamaboko
12. bamboo shoots	25. soybean sprouts	39. katsuobushi
(takenoko)	26. daizu	40. gammodoki

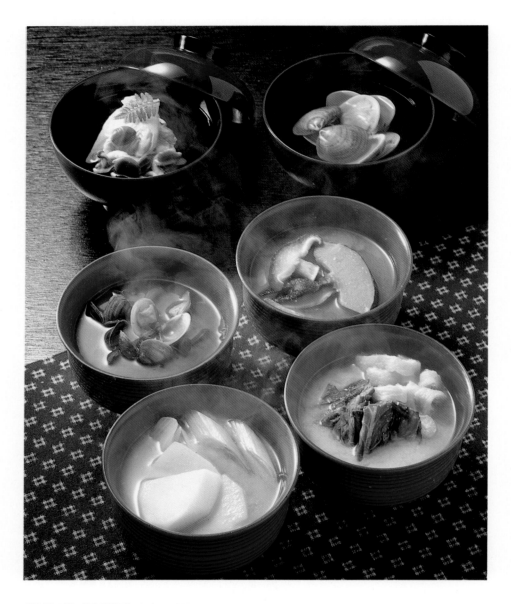

**CLEAR SOUPS (top): Chicken and shimeji (p. 113) ¤ Clam (p. 131)
MISO SOUPS: Shijimi (p. 129) ¤ Pumpkin and shiitake (p.124) ¤
Potato and green onion (p.132) ¤ Komatsuna and abura-age (p.133)**

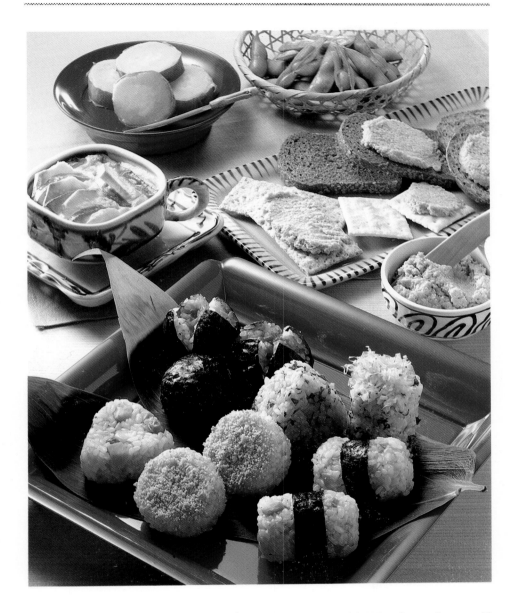

SNACKS (p. 146): Boiled sweet potatoes ¤ Boiled fresh soybeans ¤ Baked sweet potatoes and apples ¤ Soybean jam ¤ Rice balls (p. 118)

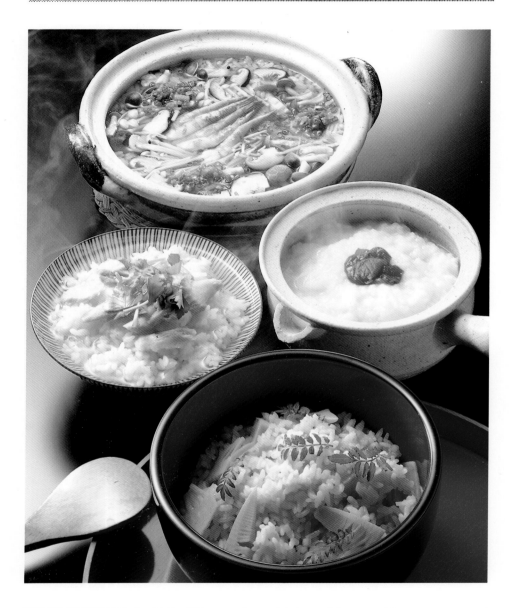

RICE DISHES (p.114): Rice and crab/vegetable porridge — zosui ¤ Salmon ochazuke (left) ¤ Rice gruel and umeboshi (right) ¤ Rice and bamboo shoots — takenoko gohan

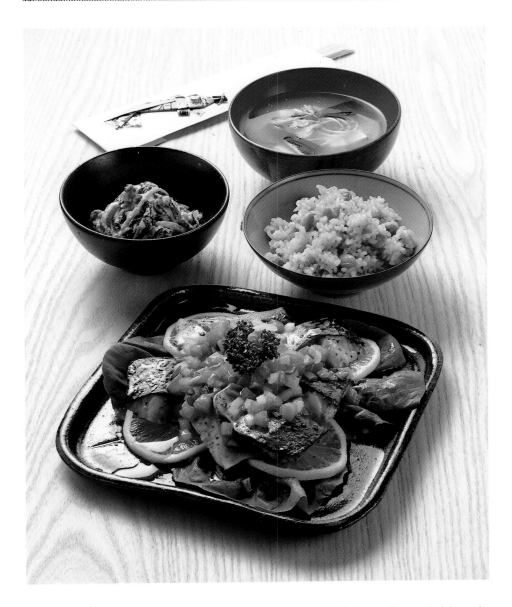

MEAL FOUR: Wakame and tofu miso soup ¤ Tofu and vegetable mix ¤ Rice ¤ Mackerel with tomato-and-onion dressing

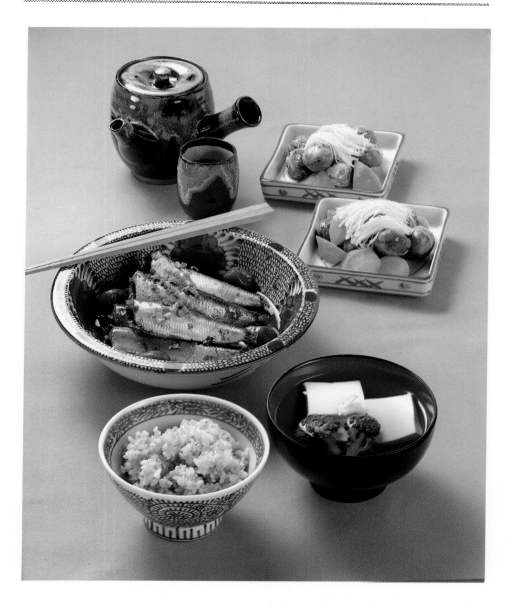

MEAL SIX: Brussel sprout and carrot salads ¤ Sardines in umeboshi sauce ¤ Rice ¤ Broccoli and tofu soup

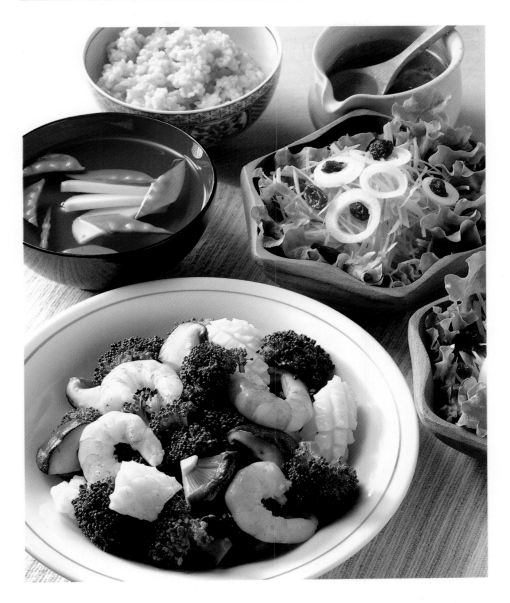

MEAL EIGHT: Rice ¤ Kamaboko and snow-pea soup ¤ Salad dressing ¤ carrot salad ¤ Shrimp, squid and broccoli

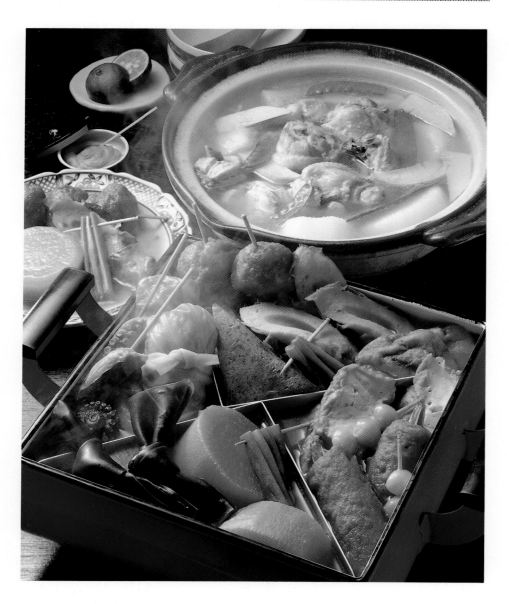

MEAL THIRTEEN: Chicken casserole
Oden (p. 138)

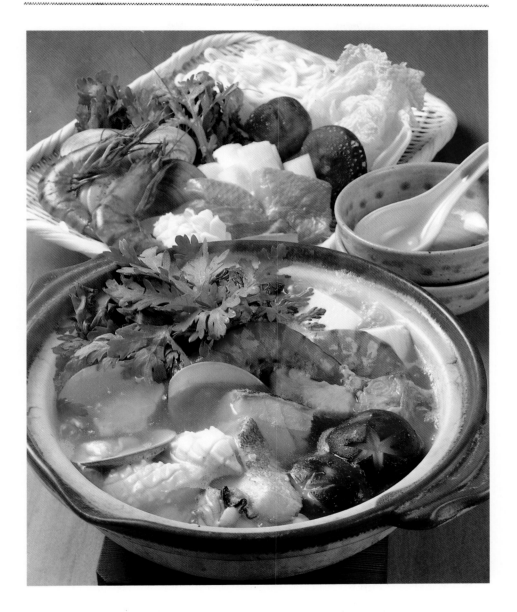

MEAL FOURTEEN: Fish casserole ingredients ¤ Fish casserole

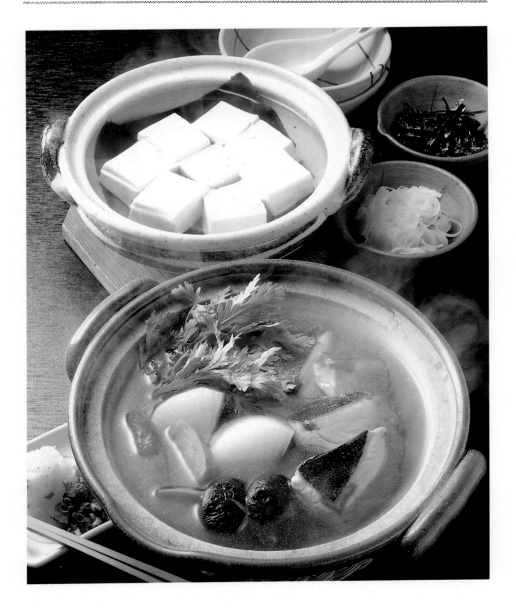

Boiled tofu and kombu (kelp) (p. 144) ¤ Nori ¤ Sliced onions ¤ Boiled Yellowtail (p. 135)

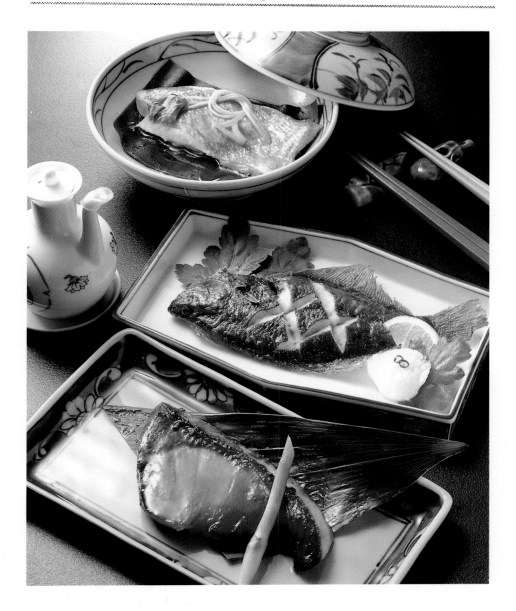

**FISH DISHES: Steamed sea bream and kombu (top) (p. 138) ¤
Boiled flatfish (middle) ¤ Yellowtail teriyaki (bottom) (p. 138)**

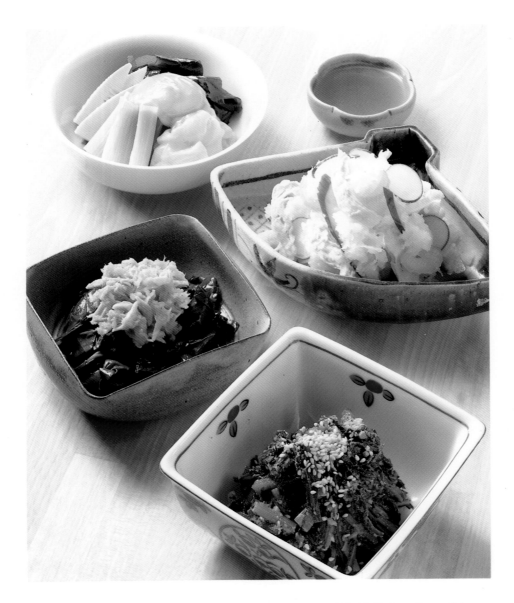

Clams and vegetables with miso dressing (p. 137) ¤ Spinach and tuna salad (p. 142) Chicken and grated daikon (p. 139) ¤ Shungiku with sesame seeds (p. 120)

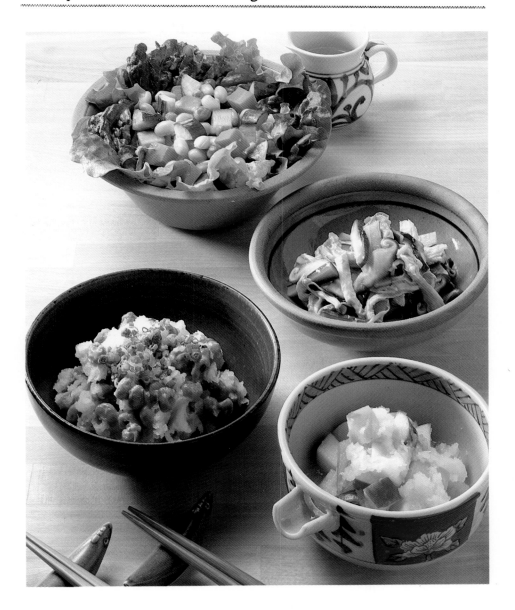

VEGETABLES DISHES: Soybean salad (p. 143) ¤ Chicken salad with vinegar dressing (p. 140) ¤ Natto mixed with grated daikon (p. 143) ¤ Vinegared fruits and vegetables salad (p. 142)

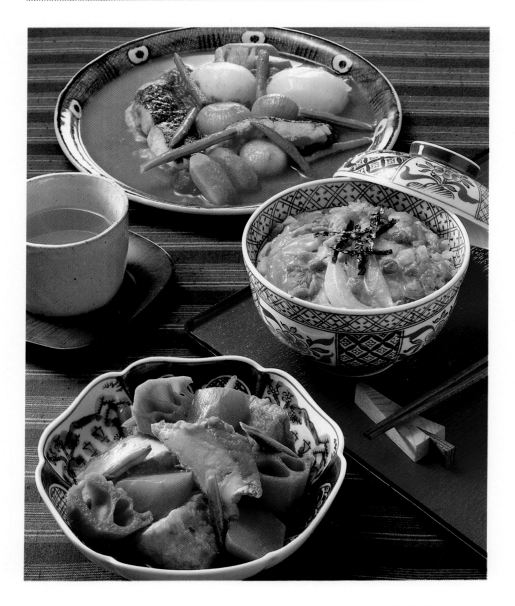

Sole stew (p. 123) ¤ Chicken and eggs on rice (p. 129) ¤ Nama-age and vegetables (p. 145)

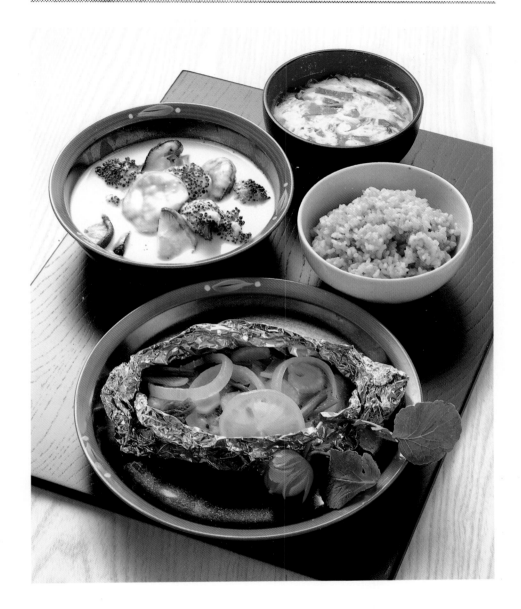

Egg and leek soup (p. 126) ¤ Creamed broccoli and mushrooms ¤ Rice ¤ Steamed chicken (p. 127)

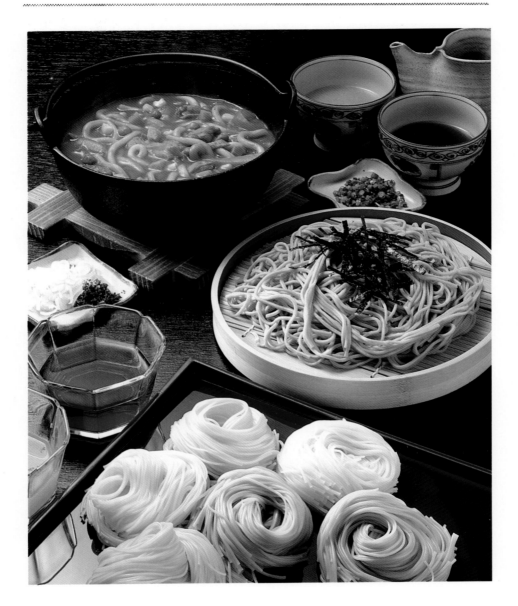

JAPANESE NOODLES (p. 148): Curry udon (top) ¤ Zaru soba (dip sauces are at top right) ¤ Somen (dip sauces are on the left)

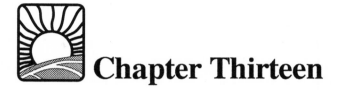

Chapter Thirteen

Recipes for the Fourteen Meals

Meal One Recipes

Wakame Soup (serves one)

Ingredients

3 oz. wakame	chopped green onions
3/4 cups of soup stock	1t of sake
4 slices bamboo shoots	a dash of salt and pepper

Directions

Rehydrate wakame and cut into 1-inch strips. Remove tough center vein if necessary. Bring stock to a boil, add bamboo shoots, sake, salt and pepper. Add wakane and green pepper. Bring to a boil and serve immediately.

61 calories; 6% fat; 35% protein; 59% carbohydrates; 0.6g sodium (per serving)

Boiled Chicken Mixed with Vegetables (serves six)

Ingredients

7 oz. skinless white chicken	10 snowpeas
7 oz. bamboo shoots	2 cups soup stock
3 carrots	1/2T salad oil
3 oz. renkon (lotus root)	3T soy sauce
1 cake konnyaku	1T mirin or dry pale sherry
4 dried shiitake mushrooms	

Directions

Cut chicken into bit-sized pieces. Peel carrots and lotus root and cut into bite-sized bits. Cut bamboo shoots and konnyaku into bite-sized pieces and boil briefly. Rehydrate mushrooms and cut into pieces. String snowpeas and boil quickly in salted water until bright green. In frying pan, heat salad oil and stir-fry chicken. Remove chicken to a dish and add soy sauce, mirin, and sugar. Add carrots, bamboo shoots, lotus root, konnyaku and mushrooms to the frying pan and stir fry. Add soup stock, sugar, soy sauce, and mirin. Simmer for 20 minutes. Add chicken and stir. Cook until water evaporates. Add snow peas and serve.

102 calories; 11% fat; 47% protein; 42% carbohydrates; 0.6g sodium (per serving)

Tofu with Daikon Leaves (serves six)

Daikon greens, the tops from long Japanese radishes, make this dish high in calcium. Turnip leaves may be substituted.

Ingredients

2 cakes of soft tofu, cut in 3/4-inch cubes

Leaves from one daikon, cut in 3/4-inch cubes

3/4-oz. shirasuboshi
2 eggs
1 cup soup stock
1T of salad oil

Directions

Briefly boil shirasuboshi. Beat eggs and add shirasuboshi. Heat salad oil in a sauce pan and stir in leaves. Add soup stock, sake, sugar and soy sauce, and bring to a boil. Add tofu and simmer over low flame. When tofu is done, pour in egg mixture and immediately turn off flame. Serve when eggs are soft boiled.

119 calories; 61% fat; 30% protein; 9% carbohydrates; 0.2g sodium (per serving)

Meal Two Recipes

Sole Stew (serves six)

Ingredients

10 oz. sole   4 turnips
12 green onions   20 string beans
2 carrots   2 medium tomatoes

Directions

Wash the sole, sprinkle with salt and pepper and lay aside.

Peel the green onions and carrots. Cut the carrots and tomatoes into bite-sized pieces. Strings the beans, cut into halves, and boil until bright green. Put the soup stock into a pot, add the carrots, onions and turnips and boil until soft. Add coarsely chopped tomatoes and simmer for 15 minutes, and then add the sole. Put in a bowl, add the string beans and serve.

70 calories; 3% fat; 55% protein; 42% carbohydrates; 0.1g sodium (per serving)

Boiled Hijiki, Carrots, and Deep-Fried Tofu Puffs (serves eight)

Ingredients

1/3 cup dried hijiki   1t sugar
2 cakes deep-fried tofu puffs   1T soy sauce
(abura-age)   1T mirin (sweet sake) or pale
 1 carrot   sherry
1/2T salad oil

Directions

Soak hijiki in water then strain, shaking off excess water. Pour boiling water over the the deep-fried tofu to reduce excess oil content and cut them and carrots into thin strips.

Heat oil in sauce pan and stir-fry carrots and deep-fried tofu.

Add hijiki to one cup of water, salt, mirin, and boil until water is absorbed. Place in serving bowl, sprinkle with sesame seeds and serve.

96 calories; 56% fat; 24% protein; 20% carbohydrates; 0.2g sodium (per serving)

Meal Three Recipes

Pumpkin and Fresh Shiitake Miso Soup (serves four)

Ingredients

2 oz. Japanese pumpkin   4 cups of soup stock
4 fresh shiitake   4T of miso

Directions

Cut the pumpkin and shiitake into 1/2-inch thick pieces. Boil the pumpkin in the soup stock. When it becomes soft, put in the miso. Finally, put in the shiitake and turn off heat.

70 calories; 10% fat; 39% protein; 51% carbohydrates; 0.4g sodium (per serving)

Chicken and Cashew Nuts (serves six)

Ingredients

2 skinned chicken breasts   3T of soup stock
3 oz. cashews   1T of salad oil
2 bell peppers, chopped   1t of soy sauce
1 small onion   2t of sake
5 oz. bamboo shoots, chopped   1T of cornstarch
1/4-inch slice ginger, chopped

Directions

Cut chicken into bite-size pieces and mix with soy sauce, sake, salt, pepper, and cornstarch. Heat oil in frying pan and stir-fry onions and ginger. Add chicken mixture and cook. Pour in soup and bring to boil. Add vegetables and cook. Add cashews and serve.

145 calories; 40% fat; 34% protein; 26% carbohydrates; 0.1g sodium (per serving)

Cauliflower Salad (serves two)

Ingredients

3 oz. cauliflower   1t salad oil
5 lettuce leaves   1t vinegar
1 hard boiled egg yolk

Directions

Boil the cauliflower until done and break into bite-sized pieces. Crumble the yolk of the egg. In a salad bowl, put in the lettuce and the cauliflower. Sprinkle the egg on top and add salad oil and vinegar dressing.

87 calories; 64% fat; 14% protein; 22% carbohydrates; 0.2g sodium (per serving)

Meal Four Recipes

Wakame and Tofu Miso Soup (serves six)

Ingredients

4 cups basic stock
5T miso (soybean paste)
1 cake soft tofu

1/3 oz. dried wakame (dry curl-ing seaweed)

Directions

Add tofu and wakame to boiling stock. Dissolve miso in a bowl with some boiling stock. Stir into soup. Heat thoroughly and serve.

64 calories; 22% fat; 39% protein; 39% carbohydrates; 0.3g sodium (per serving)

Mackerel with Tomato-and-Onion Dressing (serves eight)

Ingredients

1 lb. mackerel, cleaned
3/4 onion, chopped
2 tomatoes, chopped
1 bell pepper, chopped
parsley

2T of salad oil
1 cup of stock
1T of white wine
1T of vinegar

Directions

Salt mackeral and set aside for 10 minutes. Heat salad oil in frying pan. Add fish and pour wine and vinegar over skin. Add soup and simmer until done.

Transfer fish to serving plate and top with chopped vegetables.

185 calories; 61% fat; 30% protein; 9% carbohydrates; 0.2g sodium (per serving)

Tofu and Vegetable Mix (serves four)

Ingredients

1/3 cake of konnyaku (vegetable starch)

2 carrots, cut into matchstick-sized pieces

4T of soup stock

1T of sake

1 cake tofu

1t salt

3T sugar

1/4 cup snowpeas

3 fresh shiitake mushrooms or other mushrooms, chopped

1t of light soy sauce

1t of white miso (shiro miso soybean paste)

1t sugar

1T mirin sweet sake or pale dry sherry

2T of sesame seeds

Directions

Boil konnyaku and cut into 1-inch lengths the size of match sticks. Combine carrots and mushrooms with soup, sake, soy sauce, and sugar and boil until soft. Boil snowpeas in salted water 1/2 minute. Cut diagonally. Crush sesame seeds with mortar and pestle. Drain excess water from tofu by pressing on a slanted board. Mix tofu, sesame seeds, salt, sugar, and sake. Drain vegetables and mix with tofu.

90 calories; 32% fat; 21% protein; 47% carbohydrates; 0.8g sodium (per serving)

Meal Five Recipes

Egg and Leek Soup (serves four)

Ingredients

2 leeks

2 eggs, beaten

3 cups stock

1/2t of salt

1T of soy sauce

1/2t of sake

Directions

Cut off tough, outer green leaves, wash leeks thoroughly and cut into 1-inch strips. Boil three cups of stock, add salt, soy sauce, sake and leeks. Drizzle eggs into soup, spiraling out to the edge of the pot. Serve immediately.

65 calories; 41% fat; 46% protein; 13% carbohydrates; 0.5g sodium (per serving)

Steamed Chicken(serves one)

Ingredients

1/2 chicken breast, skinned   1 sliced clove of garlic
1/4 cup celery with leaves,   a dash of sake
sliced lengthwise into strips   juice of 1/2 lemon
1/4 onion, cut into wedges

Directions

Place chicken on a large piece of aluminium foil. Add a dash of sake. Top with vegetables. Fold foil into a package and steam in a covered steamer for 15 minutes. Open, squeeze lemon on it and serve.

(This dish can also be made with white fish. In that case sprinkle a bit of salt on the fish and let it stand for about 5 minutes. Instead of celery, onion and garlic, substitute shiitake mushrooms, and spinach.)

117 calories; 3% fat; 70% protein; 27% carbohydrates; 0.1g sodium (per serving)

Boiled Komatsuna (serves one)

Ingredients

2 oz komatsuna   1t soy sauce
1/2T white sesame seeds

Directions

Boil the komatsuna until it changes color, rinse with cold water, and squeeze out excess water. Cut to appropriate lengths and put in a bowl. Sprinkle with sesame seeds.

37 calories; 44% fat; 30% protein; 26% carbohydrates; 0.3g sodium (per serving)

Meal Six Recipes

Broccoli and Tofu Soup (serves four)

Ingredients

1 bunch broccoli, cut into bite-   3 cups of soup stock
size pieces   a pinch of salt
1/2 a cake of soft tofu, cut into   2t of soy sauce
2-inch cubes   yuzu (citron) or lemon peel,

Directions

Boil broccoli. In a sauce pan, combine stock, soy sauce and salt. Add tofu and broccoli and simmer. Serve in Japanese-style soup bowls topped with shredded citron or lemon peels.

43 calories; 23% fat; 51% protein; 26% carbohydrates; 0.2g sodium (per serving)

Sardines in Umeboshi Sauce (serves four)

Ingredients

8 fresh sardines, cleaned with heads removed
4 umeboshi (pickled plums)

4T of soy sauce
1T of sake
1t of sugar

Directions

Mix 2/3 cup of water in sauce pan with soy sauce, sake, and sugar and bring to a boil. Add sardines. When nearly done, add umeboshi. Cook over a low flame, basting sauce over sardines until the sauce has reduced by two thirds.

93 calories; 49% fat; 37% protein; 14% carbohydrates; 1.0g sodium (per serving)

Brussel Sprout and Carrot Salad(serves four)

Ingredients

12 small brussel sprouts
2 carrots, cut into bite-sized pieces
2T of light soy sauce

2T of vinegar
1T of salad oil
1/8-inch of fresh ginger, peeled and finely chopped

Directions

Cook sprouts and carrots in salted water until done. Mix soy sauce, vinegar and pour over hot vegetables, allowing flavors to blend a few minutes.

103 calories; 30% fat; 16% protein; 54% carbohydrates; 0.6g sodium (per serving)

Meal Seven Recipes

Shijimi (Fresh Water Clams) Miso Soup (serves four)

Ingredients

1 cup of shijimi   4T miso
4 cups of water

Directions

Thoroughly wash the shijimi and put in a pot. Boil until they open.
Add miso and boil until it melts and immediately turn off.
36 calories; 23% fat; 40% protein; 37% carbohydrates; 0.8g sodium (per serving)

Chicken and Eggs on Rice (serves one)

Ingredients

1/2 cup rice   2T green peas
2 oz white chicken meat   1t sugar
1 small onion   1/2T soysauce
1 egg, beaten   3T soup stock

Directions

Cut the onion into thin pieces and the chicken into bite-size cubes.
Stir fry lightly in the olive oil. Put into a sauce pan, adding the sugar
and soy sauce and soup stock and quickly bring to a boil. Drizzle in the
eggs while stirring and sprinkle the green peas on top. Put the cooked
rice in the bottom of a bowl, then top with the chicken-egg mixture.
292 calories; 20% fat; 34% protein; 46% carbohydrates; 0.1g sodium (per serving)

Vinegared Daikon and Carrots (serves four)

Ingredients

1 lb. daikon, cut into thin strips   5T of vinegar
4 carrots, cut in thin strips   1t of sugar
Juice from 1/2 lemon

Directions

Sprinkle carrots and daikon with salt and let stand. Squeeze out excess water. Add vinegar, sugar, and lemon juice. Cover with a heavy weight and let stand 30 minutes to blend flavors.

120calories; 13% fat; 11% protein; 76% carbohydrates; 0.4g sodium (per serving)

Meal Eight Recipes

Kamaboko and Snow Pea Soup (serves 4)

Ingredients

4 cm of kamaboko	2t soy sauce
12 snow peas	a dash of salt
3 cups soup stock	

Directions

Put the snow peas in boiling water for about 10 seconds, then slice each on diagonally in 3 pieces. Cut the kamaboko into 12 thin slices.

Bring stock to a boil, then add soy sauce and salt. Turn off heat.

Put snow peas and kamaboko in soup bowls and pour stock over them. It is now ready to serve.

39calories; 10% fat; 58% protein; 32% carbohydrates; 0.3g sodium (per serving)

Shrimp, Squid and Broccoli (serves two)

Ingredients

1 head of broccoli, cut into bite-sized pieces	chopped
	1-1/2T of salad oil
3 oz. squid, cut into pieces	1 cup soup stock
8 shrimps, shelled	a dash of salt and pepper
4 fresh shiitake, cut in half	1t of sugar
1/2-inch ginger, peeled and	

Directions

Boil the broccoli and drain. Heat oil in a sauce or frying pan. Stir-fry fish, mushrooms and broccoli. Add soup, sake, salt and sugar, and boil for 2 minutes. Serve.

190 calories; 51% fat; 35% protein; 14% carbohydrates; 0.1g sodium (per serving)

Carrot Salad (serves four)

Ingredients

4 large carrots, cut into thin strips
  1/2 cup raisins
  1/2 onion, sliced into thin rings

lettuce
1T soy sauce
1T vinegar

Directions

Soak raisins in hot water to plump. Combine all ingredients. Line individual bowls with lettuce leaf and top with carrot mixture.

91 calories; 0% fat; 6% protein; 94% carbohydrates; 0.5g sodium (per serving)

Meal Nine

Clam Soup (serves four)

Ingredients

12 clams
4 cups of water

1/2T of soy sauce
1/2t of salt

Directions

Thoroughly wash the clams. Boil in water on a medium flame until the clams open. Then add the soy sauce and salt. Immediately turn off flame. Don't overboil, as clams will harden.

31 calories; 12% fat; 73% protein; 15% carbohydrates; 0.4g sodium (per serving)

Boiled Chicken and Sweet Potatoes (serves three)

Ingredients

7 oz. white chicken meat
  1 sweet potato, cut into bite-sized pieces
  1/3 oz. wakame (seaweed)
  1T salad oil
  1-1/2 cups soup stock

2T sake
1t sugar
2T soy sauce
  1T mirin (sweet sake) or pale dry sherry

Directions

Rehydrate wakame and cut into bite-sized pieces. Stir fry chicken in oil. Add sweet potato and coat with oil. Add sugar, soy sauce and stock. On medium heat, cover and simmer until potatoes are done. Add sake and wakame. Boil and serve.

208 calories; 21% fat; 39% protein; 40% carbohydrates; 0.4g sodium (per serving)

Daikon, Carrots, and Cucumber Salad (serves four)

Ingredients

6 oz. daikon, cut into thin strips

2 carrots, cut into thin strips

1 cucumber, cut into strips

juice from 1/2 lemon

1T of soy sauce

1T white sesame seeds

Directions

Toss vegetables in a bowl. Top with sesame seeds and dress with lemon and soy sauce.

47 calories; 23% fat; 13% protein; 64% carbohydrates; 0.3g sodium (per serving)

Meal Ten

Potatoes and Green Onion Miso Soup (serves four)

Ingredients

1/4 lb. potatoes

1 stalk of green onion

4 cups of soup stock

4T of miso

Directions

Peel the potatoes and cut into 1/2-inch half-moon shapes. Cut the onions into 2/3-inch diagonal strips. Boil the potatoes in the soup stock. When they become soft, put in the miso. Finally, put in the onions and when the stock comes to a boil again, turn off and serve.

86 calories; 7% fat; 32% protein; 61% carbohydrates; 0.4g sodium (per serving)

Salmon Saute (serves four)

Ingredients

4 small salmon steaks   cut in half
4t flour   2 bell peppers, cut into bit-
1 egg, beaten   sized pieces
1-1/2T light margarine   1 lemon
6 fresh shiitake mushrooms,

Directions

Heat margarine in frying pan. Sprinkle the salmon with salt and pepper. Dredge in flour and dip in beaten egg. Fry salmon until done. Remove salmon and saute mushrooms and peppers in the frying pan. Serve steaks on individual plates with vegetables and lemon wedge.

167 calories; 45% fat; 42% protein; 13% carbohydrates; 0.1g sodium (per serving)

Boiled Komatsuna and Bean Sprouts (serves four)

Ingredients

1 bunch komatsuna, washed   1T vinegar
and cut into 1/2-inch lengths 1T soy sauce
6 oz. bean sprouts

Directions

Wash the bean sprouts and boil 2 to 3 minutes. Rinse immediately in cold water to cool. Boil komatsuna 2 minutes, rinse in cold water and squeeze to remove excess water. Blend vegetables with vinegar and soy sauce, then serve.

21 calories; 2% fat; 37% protein; 61% carbohydrates; 0.2g sodium (per serving)

Meal Eleven Recipes

Komatsuna and Abura-age Miso Soup (serves four)

Ingredients

1/4 bunch of komatsuna   4 cups of soup stock
1/2 sheet of abura-age   4T of miso

Directions

Thoroughly wash the komatsuna and cut into 2-inch strips. Cut the abura-age into 1/2-inch strips. Put the abura-age in a strainer and pour boiling water over it. Bring the soup stock to a boil and add the komatsuna and abura-age. Then add the miso and when it comes to a boil again turn off and serve. Don't boil the komatsuna to long!

125 calories; 45% fat; 40% protein; 15% carbohydrates; 0.8g sodium (per serving)

Chicken and Chinese Cabbage (serves four)

Ingredients

2 chicken breasts
Small-head Chinese cabbage
5 shiitake
5 oz. bamboo shoots
3T sake

1t sugar
3T soy sauce
1 thin slice ginger, chopped
1T of cornstarch
1/2T of salad oil

Directions

Rehydrate mushrooms by soaking them in hot water for 15 minutes. Cut into quarters. Cut bamboo shoots and cabbage into bite-size pieces. Cut chicken into bite-size pieces. Heat oil in saucepan and stir fry chicken. Add vegetables, sake, soy sauce, and ginger. Cook until done. Thicken with cornstarch if necessary.

131 calories; 13% fat; 45% protein; 42% carbohydrates; 0.7g sodium (per serving)

Okara (serves eight)

Ingredients

1 lb. of okara
1/2 cup green onions, cut into strips
4 oz. clams, shrimp or other shellfish, shelled

2 slices of kamaboko (fish cake) cut into strips
1/2 carrot, cut into strips
2 shiitake mushrooms

Directions

Heat oil in frying pan. Fry clams. Add vegetables and stir. Add okara. Add sake, sugar, soy sauce and cook, stirring for 2 to 3 minutes until done.

70 calories; 30% fat; 32% protein; 38% carbohydrates; 0.2g sodium (per serving)

Meal Twelve

Boiled Yellowtail (serves four)

Ingredients

4 small fillets of yellowtail tuna
cut into bite-sized pieces
1 lb daikon radish cut into half-
moon shapes 1/2 inch thick
8 shiitake mushrooms
2 carrots, cut into 1-inch cubes

4 shungiku leaves
4 cups of soup stock
2T of sake
3T of soy sauce
scallions
salt and pepper to taste

Directions

Salt fish and let stand for 5 minutes. Add to boiling water and simmer until not quite done. Remove. Cut deep crosses in the caps of the
mushrooms. Set aside. Heat soup stock, add sake, soy sauce and salt.
Add fish, radish, carrots, and mushrooms. When carrots are soft, add
shungiku. Top with grated daikon and slivered scallions and serve.
115 calories; 40% fat; 35% protein; 25% carbohydrates; 0.8g sodium (per serving)

Hijiki and Sesame Seeds (serves one)

Ingredients

1 oz. hijiki (seaweed)
1t sesame seeds
1 cup soup stock
1t of mirin or pale dry sherry

1/2t of soy sauce
1/2t of salad oil
1t sugar
dash of salt

Directions

Soak hijiki in water then strain. Heat oil in sauce pan. Stir-fry carrots and tofu. Add hijiki, soup stock, salt, sake, and boil until stock is
absorbed. Place in serving bowl, sprinkle with sesame seeds and serve.
139 calories; 23% fat; 23% protein; 54% carbohydrates; 0.5g sodium (per serving)

Meal Thirteen

Chicken Casserole (serves four)

Ingredients

3/4 lb. white chicken meat
5 leaves of Chinese cabbage,
cut into about 2-inch lengths
1 cake soft tofu cut into cubes

8 snow peas
1 oz. bamboo shoots
1 lb. daikon
one square of kombu (kelp)

Directions

Wipe the kelp with a clean towel and place at the bottom of a casserole. Top with chicken cut into bite-size pieces. Add enough water to cover the chicken and bring to a boil. When it begins to boil, remove kelp and skim foam from top of water. Lower flame and simmer for about 40 minutes, or until chicken is tender. Add tofu and vegetables and simmer until tender. Serve from casserole.

144 calories; 18% fat; 66% protein; 16% carbohydrates; 0.1g sodium (per serving)

Meal Fourteen

Fish Casserole (serves four)

Ingredients

7 oz. red snapper
4 oz. squid, cut into pieces
8 shrimps, shelled
4 clams
12 oysters
1 carrot, thinly sliced

2 scallions
5 leaves of Chinese cabbage
1 cake of soft tofu
4 shiitake mushrooms
1/4 lb. shungiku (green herb)
13 oz. udon (noodles)

Directions

In a casserole that can be used as a serving bowl, boil soup stock, adding soy sauce, sake, and thick cabbage stems. Add fish, tofu and other vegetables. When fish is done, add oysters and shrimp.

In Japan, diners pick out the food with chopsticks from the boiling stew. At the end of the meal, the udon noodles are added to the boiling stock and cooked with whatever vegetables are left.

494 calories; 9% fat; 29% protein; 62% carbohydrates; 1.6g sodium (per serving)

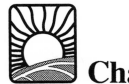 # Chapter Fourteen

Other Recipes, Snacks and Japanese Noodles

Here are some more recipes of Japanese dishes that you can try. Japanese noodles can be used for quick lunches or even for snacks.

Main Dishes (Fish)

Clams and Vegetables with Miso Dressing (serves four)

Ingredients

1/2 lb. clams (any small clam may be used)
4 green onions

bamboo shoots
1/3 oz. wakame

Ingredients for the dressing

2-1/2 oz. white miso
2t of mustard

3T of vinegar
1T of sugar

Directions

If clams are fresh, cook and loosen from shell. Drop onions in boiling water until they turn bright green and are lightly cooked. Remove, rinse in cold water and cut into 1-inch-long strips. Rehydrate wakame and cut into 1-inch strips. Boil briefly. Using only the top soft part of the bamboo shoot, cut into thin pieces and boil briefly. In a small bowl, combine mustard, vinegar, and miso topping. Arrange vegetables and clams on a platter. Top with mustard mixture.

101 calories; 9% fat; 35% protein; 56% carbohydrates; 0.9g sodium (per serving)

Steamed Seabream and Kombu (serves one)

Ingredients
4 oz. seabream or any other firm, white fish

1 sheet of kombu (seaweed)

3 long stems of mitsuba (trefoil), with leaves

yuzu (citron) or lemon peel

Directions
Wipe kombu with towel and place in bottom of bowl. Season fish with salt and sake, and steam for about 15 minutes. During last 5 minutes of steaming, add mitsuba and yuzu peel.

155 calories; 22% fat; 62% protein; 16% carbohydrates; 0.1g sodium (per serving)

Yellowtail Teriyaki (serves four)

Ingredients
4 pieces of yellowtail tuna

4T soy sauce

4T mirin (sweet sake) or dry

pale sherry

2-3T of sugar

Directions
In a small sauce pan, bring soy, mirin and sugar to a boil. Turn off heat. Bake the fish. When it begins to change color, baste with sauce and turn. Repeat, turning fish twice.

106 calories; 51% fat; 33% protein; 16% carbohydrates; 0.9g sodium (per serving)

Oden (serves four)

This is a nutritious, popular casserole often served in the cool autumn months. Like most casseroles it is a meal in itself. A hard boiled egg with the shell removed is often added. It is not necessary to use all the ingredients listed below, six to ten will do. Most of the ingredients can be purchased already packaged.

Ingredients
2 cakes nama-age

1 cake of konnyaku

16 string beans

8 inches of a daikon

12 ginkgo nuts

4 strips of kombu (kelp)

4 cabbage leaves

1 chikuwa (fish paste rolls)

4 satsuma-age balls

4 shrimps wrapped in abura-
age

4 octopus tentacles

7 cups of stock

1/3 cup of light soy sauce

2T of sugar

3T of mirin

Ingredients for the cabbage roll

4 leaves of Chinese cabbage

3 oz. ground white chicken

2 T chopped onions

2T chopped bamboo shoots

Directions

Tie the kombu strips in knots and place at the bottom of a caserole. Add soup stock and bring to a boil. Just as it is about to come to a boil reduce to a low flame and add the sugar, soy sauce, and mirin, followed by the vegetables and konnyaku. Bring to a boil again over high flame, but reduce to low flame and let it simmer for for about 10 minutes. Add the tofu products and bring to a boil, immediately reducing to a low flame. Finally, add the fish and meat products and let it simmer over a low flame with the lid on the casserole for about an hour. The diners help themselves from the casserole.

To make the cabbage rolls, mix the ground chicken, onions, and bamboo shoots together. Dip the cabbage leaves in boiling water to soften, then wrap the chicken mix with the leaves. Tie with kampyo (groud shavings) or simply with a string.

Calorie and nutrient counts are not given since not all the ingredients above will be used. However, if you use the nama-age, satsuma-age and abura-age, be sure to reduce their oil content by putting them in a strainer and pouring boiling water over them.

Main Dishes (Chicken)

Chicken and Grated Daikon (serves four)

Ingredients

1 lb. daikon radish

1 cucumber

1 stalk of celery

3 radishes

1/2 lb. skinned chicken breasts

one lemon

1T of soy sauce

Directions

Salt chicken and season with sake. Steam until tender. Cool and tear into bite-sized pieces. Grate daikon and drain out excess water. Cut celery and cucumber into thin slices. Combine radish, celery and cucumber with chicken in a bowl.

Make the dressing by combining soy sauce and lemon juice. Serve dressing in individual bowls. Guests take chicken from the serving bowl and add their own dressing.

97 calories; 11% fat; 59% protein; 30% carbohydrates; 0.3g sodium (per serving)

Chicken Salad with Vinegar Dressing (serves four)

Ingredients

4 oz white chicken meat	a dash of salt
1 large cucumber	1/2t cornstarch
1 fresh shiitake mushroom	1/2t of soy sauce
1T vinegar	1T of soup stock
a dash of sugar	

Directions

Steam the chicken breasts until done and shred into small pieces. Cut the shiitake into small pieces and boil in some soup stock. Cut the cucumbers into thin, 1-inch lengths, dunk them into salted water and squeeze off excess water. Mix with dressing and put in a serving bowl. To make dressing, mix equal amounts of vinegar and soup stock with sugar salt and soy sauce. Put in a sauce pan and bring to a boil, then simmer over a low flame adding cornstarch while mixing. Immediately turn off flame.

44 calories; 3% fat; 67% protein; 30% carbohydrates; 0.1g sodium (per serving)

Side Dishes

Brussel Sprouts with Mustard Dressing (serves one)

Ingredients

50 grams brussel sprouts	1t of soy sauce
A dab of mustard	

Directions

Boil the brussel sprouts until they turn dark green. Mix the mustard and soy sauce together and add to the brussel sprouts.

33 calories; 10% fat; 23% protein; 67% carbohydrates; 0.3g sodium (per serving)

Daikon Salad (serves four)

Ingredients

6 oz. daikon radish	4T of lemon juice
5 oz. carrots	2T of soy sauce

Directions

Cut daikon and carrots into thin strips. Toss with lemon and soy sauce.

31 calories; 9% fat; 16% protein; 75% carbohydrates; 0.6g sodium (per serving)

Spinach and Bean Sprouts Sauteed (serves four)

Ingredients

1 bunch spinach	1T of salad oil
3/4 lb. bean sprouts	salt and pepper

Directions

Cut spinach into 2-inch pieces and boil for 2 minutes. Plunge into cold water, drain and squeeze out the water. Wash the bean sprouts and shake off excess water. Heat oil in a frying pan and stir fry the bean sprouts and spinach. Add salt and pepper.

45 calories; 28% fat; 26% protein; 46% carbohydrates; 0.1g sodium (per serving)

Spinach and Bonito Flakes (serves two)

Ingredients

1 bunch spinach	1t of soy sauce
bonito flakes	

Directions

Boil spinach until it darkens (less than a minute). Rinse with cold water. Trim to 1-1/2 inch portions and squeeze out excess water by hand. Place in saucer, sprinkle with bonito flakes and soy sauce. Serve.

9 calories; 0% fat; 50% protein; 50% carbohydrates; 0.2g sodium (per serving)

Spinach and Tuna Salad (serves four)

Ingredients

1 bunch spinach   1t of soy sauce
1 can tuna

Directions

Boil the spinach for one minute. Rinse with cold water and cut into 1-1/2-inch lengths. Squeeze out excess water. Add tuna and mix. Dress with soy sauce.

72 calories; 6% fat; 89% protein; 5% carbohydrates; 0.3g sodium (per serving)

Vinegared Fruits and Vegetable Salad (serves four)

Ingredients

2 oz. daikon, grated   1/2 cucumber
1 persimmon (or any other   2t vinegar
firm fruit)   1t sugar
1 apple   a pinch of salt

Directions

Mix the grated daikon with the vinegar, sugar and salt. Peel the apple, persimmon and cucumber, and cut into bite-sized pieces. Mix everything together and serve.

98 calories; 2% fat; 1% protein; 97% carbohydrates; 0.1g sodium (per serving)

Soybean Dishes

Boiled Soybeans, Shiitake and Carrots (serves four)

This is a high-nutrient, low-calorie, yet filling dish. The dried soybeans must be soaked in water for about 10 hours before cooking.

Ingredients

3-1/2 oz. soaked, dried   4 dried shiitake mushrooms
soybeans   2 cups soup stock
1/3 cake of konnyaku   1 T of sugar
3 carrots   6 T of soy sauce
one 4-inch strip kombu   3 T of sake

Directions

Boil soaked soybeans until soft. Drain and set aside. Dice kon-nyaku, kombu, carrots, and mushrooms into small cubes about the size of beans. Put vegetables and beans in boiling soup stock and cook over moderate flame. Add soy sauce, sugar, and sake, and serve.

168 calories; 23% fat; 32% protein; 45% carbohydrates; 1.5g sodium (per serving)

Natto (Fermented Soybeans) Mixed with Grated Daikon (serves one)

Ingredients

1 oz natto (fermented soybeans)	2T chopped onions
	1t soy sauce
2 oz. grated daikon	

Directions

Mix the natto with daikon and onions, adding soy sauce.

72 calories; 12% fat; 73% protein; 15% carbohydrates; 1.8g sodium (per serving)

Soybean Salad (serves four)

Ingredients

4 oz. soybeans	2 leaves lettuce
1 carrot	1T olive oil
30 green peas	1T vinegar
1 cucumber	salt and pepper

Directions

Soak the soy beans overnight and boil until tender. Cut the cucumber into 1/3-inch strips and set aside. Cut the carrots into 1/3-inch cubes, boil until tender and set aside. Boil the green peas until done and set aside. Mix vegetables with the olive oil and vinegar, adding salt and pepper. Line a bowl with lettuce and place the vegetables on top. Serve.

81 calories; 39% fat; 21% protein; 40% carbohydrates; 0.1g sodium (per serving)

Tofu Dishes

Boiled Tofu and Kombu
(serves four)

Ingredients

3 cakes tofu

6-inch square of kombu (kelp)

1/3 cup stock

1/3 cup mirin (sweet sake) or

pale dry sherry

2/3 cup soy sauce

a small chunk of ginger, grated

1/3 onion

Directions

Cut tofu into 2-inch cubes. Snip kombu at the sides in 2 or 3 places. Cut onion into thin strips. Mix the stock, mirin, the soy sauce, and ginger and bring to a boil in a saucepan. In a ceramic casserole, place the kombu on the bottom, add a small amount of water and tofu. When the mixture boils, add stock mixture from the saucepan. Simmer.

126 calories; 30% fat; 29% protein; 41% carbohydrates; 1.1g sodium (per serving)

Gammodoki, Shiitake and Vegetables
(serves four)

Ingredients

12 small gammodoki

8 shiitake or other mushrooms

12 string beans

2-1/2 cups stock

4T sugar

3T soy sauce

2T mirin

Directions

In a strainer, pour boiling water on each side of the gammodoki to reduce excess oil content. In a sauce pan bring stock to a boil. Add mushrooms and gammodoki. Add sugar, sake, soy sauce, and heat to blend flavors. Add string beans and simmer until done.

143 calories; 37% fat; 35% protein; 28% carbohydrates; 0.8g sodium (per serving)

Nama-age and eggs
(serves one)

Ingredients

40 grams nama-age (deep fried tofu cutlets)
1 small onion
1 carrot
10 snow peas

1/2 cup of soup stock
one egg, beaten
1t of soy sauce
1t sugar
a pinch of salt

Directions

In a strainer, pour boiling water over each side of the nama-age to reduce excess oil content. Cut the nama-age in bite-size cubes. Cut the carrots into 1-inch lengths. Cut onions into rings. Cut the snow peas diagonally and remove strings. Bring the stock to a boil with the onions and carrots. Add nama-age to the boiling stock and add salt and sugar. Finally, add the snow peas and drizzle the eggs into the boiling stock. Serve.

161 calories; 54% fat; 31% protein; 15% carbohydrates; 0.4g sodium (per serving)

Nama-Age and Vegetables
(serves two)

Ingredients

4 oz nama-age
3 oz lotus roots
1 carrots
5 string beans

1t sugar
1t soy sauce
a pinch of salt

Directions

In a strainer, pour boiling water over each side of the nama-age to reduce oil content. Cut the nama-age, lotus roots, carrots into bite-sized pieces, and the string beans diagonally. Boil for 15 minutes with sugar, soy sauce and salt.

113 calories; 23% fat; 24% protein; 53% carbohydrates; 0.3g sodium (per serving)

Snacks

Boiled Fresh Soybeans (Edamame) (serves four)

Ingredients
1/3 lb. fresh soybeans   a dash of salt

Directions
Fill a large pot with water and boil. Add salt and boil the fresh soybeans in the pods over a high flame for 5 to 7 minutes. If the beans are frozen, boil for only 3 to 5 minutes.
108 calories; 40% fat; 35% protein; 26% carbohydrates; 0.0g sodium (per serving)

Soybean Jam

Ingredients
one cup of fresh soybeans   1t of sugar
without the pods   a dash of salt
1/5 cup of low-fat milk

Directions
After boiling the soybeans take off the pods. Mash them. Mix with the milk, sugar and salt.
Note. The edamame will deteriorate very quickly, so don't store for more than two days. When storing, be sure to refrigerate.
365 calories (for all ingredients); 37% fat; 32% protein; 31% carbohydrates; 0.0g sodium (one serving equals 1 tablespoon)

Boiled Sweet Potatoes (serves one)

Ingredients
1/3 lb. sweet potatoes   a dash of salt
2/3 cups of water   1T mirin
1t of sugar

Directions

Thoroughly wash the sweet potatoes. Cut into 2/3-inch disks but do not peel. Carefully place them in the bottom of a pan, and add water, sugar, and salt. Turn on heat to medium flame and boil (about 10 minutes). When the potatoes are cooked put in the mirin. Continue boiling until the water is nearly gone.

191 calories; 0% fat; 5% protein; 95% carbohydrates; 0.1g sodium (per serving)

Baked Sweet Potatoes and Apples (serves four)

Ingredients

1 lb. sweet potatoes	1 egg
2 apples	1 cup low-fat milk
1T flour	1/4t vanilla flavor
1t sugar	a dash of cinnamon
1/2t salt	2t of butter

Directions

Peel the sweet potatoes and cut into 1/2-inch disks. Cut the apples into half-wedges. Soak the apples in lightly salted water for 5 minutes, remove from water and drain. Spread butter in a pyrex or ceramic dish for baking. In a separate bowl, make the dressing by thoroughly mixing the flour, sugar, salt, egg and milk. Add the vanilla flavor and cinnamon. Fill the baking dish, laying the apples and potatoes alternately. Pour the dressing over the apples and potatoes. Bake in the oven for 20 to 30 minutes at 200 degrees centigrade.

190 calories; 17% fat; 11% protein; 72% carbohydrates; 0.1g sodium (per serving)

Japanese Noodles

Japanese noodles can make for a nutritious low-calorie lunch or snack. There are many varieties available, but soba, udon and somen are the most common. Below are some representative recipes.

Zaru Soba (serves eight)

Ingredients

3/4 lb. packaged soba
1/2 sheet of slightly singed nori
chopped green onions

a dab of wasabi
red pepper

Directions

Boil the soba until tender, but don't overcook. Rinse in cold water and put on a plate. Prepare a small saucer for the green onions and wasabi. These should be mixed into the dip sauce by the diner.
151 calories; 6% fat; 15% protein; 79% carbohydrates; 0.0g sodium (per serving)

When making zaru soba, the important thing is the dip sauce that goes with it. This is what gives the soba its taste and flavor. Following are two different sauces that you might like to try. Bear in mind, however, that much of the dips are not eaten. Some is left over in the saucer and some of it left in the plate. For this reason, the calories and salt content of what is actually eaten is usually much less than given here.

Soba Dip Sauce (Tsuyu)

Ingredients

2 cups of soup stock
3T mirin

1t sugar
1/2 cup soy sauce

Directions

Bring the soup stock to a boil, mix in the mirin, and let it cool.
44 calories; 2% fat; 35% protein; 63% carbohydrates; 1.7g sodium (per serving)

Miso Dip Sauce (Tsuyu)

Ingredients
2 cups of soup stock
2T sesame seeds
4T miso
2T mirin

chopped green onions
a dab of wasabi
red pepper

Directions
Stir fry the sesame seeds and crush. Mix with the miso while adding the soup stock. Add mirin and thoroughly mix.

76 calories; 26% fat; 25% protein; 49% carbohydrates; 0.4g sodium (per serving)

Curry Udon (serves one)

The Japanese often eat curry, although the kind sold in Japan is not as hot as some would like it. Curry rice is a perennial favorite. The dish below, using udon, gives a tasty, low-calorie lunch that can be prepared in a jiffy.

Ingredients
1/4 lb. packaged udon
4 oz. of thinly cut white chick-
ed meat
1/4 of an onion
1T of peas
2-inch stalk of green onion

1T of salad oil
1-1/2 cups of soup stock
1-1/2t of curry powder
a dash of salt
2T of cornstarch

Directions
Boil the udon in 4 cups of water. When tender, leave it turn off and leave in to keep it warm.

Put the salad oil in a frypan and stir fry the chicken, onions, and peas. Add the soup stock, followed by the curry powder and salt. Mix the cornstarch with 1T of water and add to thicken curry soup.

Shake the udon dry, put in a bowl, pour the curry soup over it, and serve.

507 calories; 10% fat; 16% protein; 74% carbohydrates; 0.6g sodium (per serving)

Somen (serves eight)

Directions
Put a pound of somen in a big pot of boiling water and boil for 2 minutes. Add 1/2 cup of water and wait until it comes to a boil again.
206 calories; 19% fat; 10% protein; 71% carbohydrates; 0.7g sodium (per serving)

Somen Dip Sauce

Ingredients
2 cups of soup stock   chopped green onions
3T mirin   wasabi
2t sugar   grated ginger
1/2T soy sauce

Directions
Bring the soup stock to a boil and add the mirin, sugar and soy sauce. Let cool.
29 calories; 3% fat; 28% protein; 69% carbohydrates; 0.1g sodium (per serving)

Chicken Soup Dip Sauce

Ingredients
2 cups of soup stock made   a dash of pepper
from chicken bones   chopped parsley and celery
2 bouillon cubes

Directions
Bring to a boil, add bouillon cubes, pepper, celery, and parsley. Let cool and serve.
20 calories; 26% fat; 56% protein; 18% carbohydrates; 0.5g sodium (per serving)

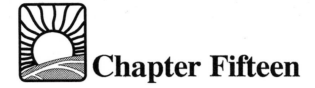

Chapter Fifteen

Japanese Food Ingredients

Before you can start preparing Japanese dishes, you are going to have to stock your kitchen with the necessary ingredients. All the ingredients that are contained in the recipes in this book are listed here and are available throughout the United States. Some you will be able to find at any supermarket, while others can be found in health-food stores. In the end you will probably have to become a regular customer of your nearest Oriental food store. Fortunately, there are many such stores, and you will find a listing of them in the appendix.

Vegetables

Bamboo shoots — These are found in many Japanese dishes and often are part of boiled or stir-fried mixed vegetables.

Chinese Cabbage — This vegetable is used mainly in one-pot dishes such as fish casserole. It is also called *hakusai* or *napa*.

Daikon (Japanese radish) — A white radish about 18 inches long or longer.

Enokidake Mushrooms — These crisp and aromatic mushrooms are a common ingredient in soups and sukiyaki.

Japanese Pumpkin — Japanese pumpkin (*kabocha*) is not the orange type used during Halloween. It is green and similar to squash.

Kampyo — Strips of dried, edible gourd used for tying food. Before use, they must be soaked in salt water, rinsed, and boiled until soft.

Komatsuna — A green leafy vegetable, extremely high in calcium. (*Brassica rapa*)

Konnyaku — Konnyaku is a jellied paste, with a high calcium content, made from the tuberous root of the *devil's tongue*. It is usually sold in 3-inch square blocks and consists of about 97% water. While tasteless, it absorbs the flavors of other foods.

Lotus Root — Long used as a folk medicine in Japan, lotus roots have a crisp texture and are excellent when boiled with other vegetables like carrots and kelp.

Shiitake — A popular mushroom in Japan. Contains substances reported to inhibit growth of tumors and to lower blood cholesterol.

Shimeji — Champignon or meadow mushrooms (*Lyophyllum aggregatum*).

Shirataki — Konnyaku in long thin strips. Often served with beef dishes like sukiyaki.

Shiso — A mint-like leaf from the beefsteak plant. Used as a garnish in many Japanese dishes and to accompany raw fish.

Shungiku (chrysanthemum leaves) — These leaves are boiled like spinach and are a standard vegatable in one-pot dishes. They are not the leaf of the commonly grown flower!

Trefoil (*mitsuba*) — Green leaves used as a garnish.

Yuzu — A small citrus fruit, the peels of which are used as a garnish in many Japanese soups dishes.

Seaweeds

Kombu (kelp) — The basic ingredient for making soup stock. It is also used in many one-pot dishes. *Kombu* has a natural white covering which should not be washed off. Instead, wipe it with a damp towel, then soak it in lukewarm water until it increases to about twice its original size.

Hijiki — *Hijiki* has the highest calcium content of all seaweeds and is also high in iron. A serving of 50 grams will supply you with more than 100% of your daily calcium and iron requirements. Often served in a small dish with carrot slivers or peas.

Nori — Seaweed strips. Also known as 'laver'. Best known in the West for its use in making *sushi*. Extremely high in vitamins and minerals.

Wakame — Ideal for salads and Japanese soups. The salt can be removed by soaking it in cold water. Before use, it should be soaked in warm water until it doubles in size.

Soybeans and Soybean Products

Abura-age — See *Deep-Fried Tofu Puffs.*

Atsu-age — See *Deep-Fried Tofu Cutlets.*

Daizu — Soybeans

Deep-Fried Tofu Cutlets (*nama-age* or *atsu-age*) — Cakes of tofu, deep fried.

Deep-Fried Tofu Puffs (*abura-age*) — Thin puffs of tofu, deep fried.

Dried Soybeans — Mature dried soybeans are available packaged throughout the U.S.

Edamame — See *Fresh Green Soybeans*.

Fresh Green Soybeans (*edamame*) — Fresh soybeans boiled in the pods.

Freeze-Dried Tofu — Frozen and dried tofu cakes.

Gammodoki — Deep-fried tofu patties with thinly diced vegetables, sesame seeds, and seaweed.

Grilled Tofu (*yaki-dofu*) — Pressed and grilled tofu.

Okara — The residue of crushed soybeans which have been used to make tofu.

Miso — Fermented soybean paste. There are two types: white miso, which is actually a light creamy yellow, and red miso which is brown. Besides being used in soup, it is also used as a dressing or as a dip for vegetable dishes.

Nama-Age — See *Deep-Fried Tofu Cutlets*.

Natto — Whole fermented soybeans. Often eaten with rice for breakfast.

Soybean Sprouts — Four- to five-day-old sprouting soybeans.

Tofu — Tofu (bean curd) comes in two main varieties: cotton (or firm) tofu and silk (or soft) tofu.

Yaki-Dofu — See *Grilled Tofu*.

Noodles

Soba — Long, brown, thin noodles made from buckwheat flour mixed with unbleached wheat flour. The amount of buckwheat in soba ranges from 40% to 100%.

Somen — Thin, white noodles made from wheat flour.

Udon — Thick, round, white noodles made from wheat flour.

Fish and Fish Products

Bonito Flakes — Made from the shavings of dried bonito. They are used as a base for soup stocks and sprinkled over boiled vegetables.

Chikuwa — Ground white-fish meat made into a paste and either steamed or grilled. They are molded into about 6-inch long rings.

Kamaboko — Ground white-fish meat made into a paste and formed into 6-inch cakes.

Katsuobushi — See *Bonito Flakes*

Satsuma-age Balls — Balls of deep\fried kamaboko.

Shijimi — Fresh water clams.

Shirasuboshi — Dried young sardines. Also called "whitebait".

Condiments

Dashi no moto — Packaged soup stock

Mirin — A sweet syrupy rice wine (*sake*) used in many Japanese dishes.

Rice Vinegar — Sweeter than western vinegar. Made from white rice. It softens hard vegetables during cooking

Sake — Japan's traditional 'wine'. It is made from steamed rice and a mold called *koji*. Although an alcoholic beverage, it is also an essential ingredient in many Japanese dishes.

Sesame Seeds — Sesame seeds (*goma*) are used as a garnish in many Japanese dishes. For the best use of their nutrients, they should be toasted and then ground. They come in two varieties: white and black seeds. Both are extremely high in calcium and magnesium.

Soy Sauce — The main seasoning used with Japanese foods.

Umeboshi — Made from unripe plums which are soaked in brine along with shiso leaves.

Wasabi — Japanese horseradish. A sharp-tasting green paste used on sushi and other dishes.

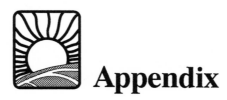

Appendix

Suppliers of Japanese Foods

If your local supermarket doesn't stock some of the foods listed in this book, you should be able to find them at oriental, health, or natural food stores. Gourmet shops also carry many Japanese foods.

The following list includes some other sources. Some of these firms sell food by mail. The importers and manufacturers on the list generally do not sell food directly, but they can give you the names of retailers in your area who carry their products.

Arkansas

Mountain Ark Trading Co.
120 S. East Street
Fayetteville, AR 72701
(800) 643-8909
Mail order

California

House of Rice
338 Broadway
Chico, CA 95928
(916) 893-1794
Retail

Japan Food Corporation
445 Kaufman Court
San Francisco, CA 94080
(415) 873-8400. Importer

Japantown Foods
5289-F Prospect Rd.
San Jose, CA 95129
(408) 255-7980. Retail

Nishimoto Trading Co., Ltd.
1111 Mateo St.
Los Angeles, CA 90021
(213) 689-9330. Importer

Nishimoto Trading Co., Ltd.
410 East Grand Ave.,
South San Francisco, CA 94080
(415) 871-2490. Importer

Ohsawa America
P.O. Box 12717,
Northgate Station
San Rafael, CA 94913
(800) 647-2929. Importer

San-J International
384 Liberty
San Francisco, CA 94114
(415) 821-4040
Manufacturer

Westbrae Natural Foods
4240 Hollis Street
Emeryville, CA 94608
(213) 722-1692
Manufacturer

Colorado

East-West Gifts
203 West Myrtle
Fort Collins, CO 80521
(303) 493-0808. Mail order

Florida

Tree of Life, Inc.
PO Box 410
St. Augustine, FL 32084
(904) 824-8181
Manufacturer

Illinois

Toguri Mercantile Co.
851 W. Belmont Ave.
Chicago, IL 60657
(312) 929-3500
Retail

Maryland

Sakura Oriental Books and
Food
15809 South Frederick Rd.
Rockville, MD 20855
(301) 468-0605
Retail

Michigan

Eden Foods
701 Tecumseh Rd.
Clinton, MI 49236
(517) 456-7424
Importer, ask for customer ser-
vice

New Jersey

Edward & Sons
Box 3150
Union, NJ 07083
(201) 964-8176
Importer

Nishimoto Trading Co., Ltd.
21-23 Empire Blvd.
South Hackensack, NJ 07606
(212) 349-0056. Importer

Nebraska

Aki Oriental Foods & Gifts
4425 So. 84th Street
Omaha, NE 68127
(402)339-2671
Retail

New York

The Kimms
316 Wall Street
Kingston, NY 12401
(914) 331-3999
Retail

Oregon

Anzen Pacific Corp.
P.O Box 11407
Portland, OR 97211
(503) 283-1284
Retail, mail order

Import Plaza
#1 N.W. Couch St.
Portland, OR 97209
(503) 227-4050. Retail
21 stores throughout Oregon

Washington

Granum
2901 NE Blakely St.
Seattle, WA 98105
(206) 525-0051
Retail, mail order

Uwajimaya
6th So. & So. King
Seattle, WA 98104
(206) 624-6248
Retail 3 stores, mail order

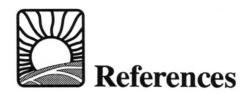 **References**

This book is not meant to be a scientific treatise. Consequently, we have not given footnotes in the text nor have we documented many of the scientific statements made there. However, all these statements are based on the results of experiments and investigations reported in reputable scientific publications by scientists working in the field of obesity and related subjects. For those interested in reading this literature, a partial list of the most important publications we referred to while writing this book are given.

References to Chapter One

Van Itallie TB, Yang MU (1984): *Cardiac dysfunction in obese dieters: a potentially lethal complication of rapid, massive weight loss*. American Journal of Clinical Nutrition **39**, 695.

Russel D, *et al* (1984): *Metabolic and structural changes in skeletal muscle during hypocaloric dieting*. American Journal of Clinical Nutrition. **39** 503.

Dore C, Hesp R, Wilkins D & Garrow JS. (1982): *Prediction of energy requirements of obese patients after massive weight loss*. Hum. Nutr.: Clin. Nutr. **36C**, 41–48.

Keys A, Brozek J, Hanschel A *et. al.* (1950): *The biology of human starvation*. Minneapolis: University of Minnesota Press.

References to Chapter Two

Morales G, Rocco ME: *Sistema de informacion, medicion y prediccion de estado de nutricion del sector obrero*. First Venezuelan Congress of Nutrition, Caracas (1985). Abstract #63.

Richards R, de Caceres M: *The problem of obesity in developing countries: its prevalence and morbidity*. In Obesity (1974). Burland, Samuel, Yudkin eds. London: Churchill Livingstone.

Fallon AE, Rozin P (1985): *Sex differences in perception of desirable body shape.* Journal of Abnormal Psychology. **94**, 102–105.

Pugliese HT, Lifschitz F, Grod G, *et. al.* (1983): *Fear of obesity: a cause of short stature and delayed puberty.* New England Journal of Medicine, **309**, 513.

Starvaholics? Anorexics may be addicted to a starvation "high". Scientific American, November 1988. Page 21

Greenwood MRC: *Normal and abnormal growth and maintainance of adipose tissue.* Recent Advances in Obesity Research: IV. John Libbey, London/Paris. 20–25.

References to Chapter Three

Sims EAH (1976): *Experimental obesity, dietary-induced thermogenesis, and their clinical implications.* Clinical Endocrinology and Metabolism **5**, 377–395.

Benditt EP: *The origin of atherosclerosis.* Scientific American, February 1977, 74–85.

Cohen LA: *Diet and cancer.* Scientific American November 1987, 42–48.

(According to Japan's Health and Welfare Ministry the daily average salt intake in Japan as of 1988 was 11.7 grams. In southwestern Japan the average ranges from 6.2 to 10.5 grams a day. Average US intake is reported to be a bit over 12 grams a day.)

(Are all calories are equal? Fatty foods have the greatest potential to be stored as fat in the body. Refer to the following paper.)
Schiemann R, Nehring K, Hoffmann L *et. al.* (1971): *Energetische Futterbewertung und Energienormen.* Berlin: VEB Deutscher Landwirtschaftsverlag.

References for Chapter Four

Cohen LA: *Diet and cancer.* Scientific American. November 1987; 42–48

Lands WEM: *Fish and human health* (1986). Academic Press.

Dietary fibre and obesity. International Journal of Obesity (1987), Vol. 11 #1.

References for Chapter Five

Neumann RO (1902): *Experimentalle Beitrag zur Lehre von dem taglichen Nahrungsbedarf des Menschen unter besonderer Berucksichtigung der notwendigen Eiweissmenge.* Arch. Hyg. **45**, 1–87.

Miller DS, Mumford P, Stock MJ (1967): *Gluttony II: Thermogenesis in overeating man.* American Journal Clinical Nutrition, **20**, 1223–1229.

Bondy PK, Rosenberg LE (1980): *Metabolic Control and Disease.* W.B. Saunders Company

Berchtold P, Van Itallie TB(1985): *Physiological prognostic factors for the treatment of obesity.* Recent Advances in Obesity Research: IV. John Libbey, London/Paris, 320–325.

Cormillot A, Fuchs A, Zuckerfeld: *A network for multifaceted treatment of obesity based on the addictive behavioral model.* (1985) Recent Advances in Obesity Research: IV. John Libbey, London/Paris, 375–382.

Wurtman RJ, Wurtman JJ: *Carbohydrates and depression.* Scientific American, January 1989, 50–57.

References for Chapter Six

Berger M, Kemmer FW, Becker K, *et. al. Effect of physical training on glucose tolerance and on glucose metabolism of skeletal muscles in anaesthetised normal rats.* Diabetologia **16**, 179–184.

Krotkiewski M: *Physical training in obesity with varying degree of glucose intolerance.* The Journal of Obesity and Weight Regulation, Fall 1985, 179–206.

Suzuki M (1985): *Hyaku sai no kagaku* (The science of centenarians), Shinkosensho, Tokyo.

Lithell H, Cedermark M, Fröberg J, *et. al.* (1981): *Increase in lipoprotein-lipase activity in skeletal muscle during heavy exercise. Relation to epinephrine excretion.* Metabolism **30**, 1130–1134.

References for Chapter Seven

Rebuffé-Scrive M (1987): *Regional adipose tissue metabolism in women during and after reproductive life and in men.* Recent Advances in Obesity Research: V. John Libbey, London/Paris, 82–91.

Index

Make it easy to follow a
balanced, low-fat diet with the

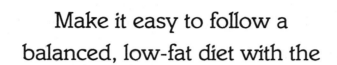

East Meets West
Nutrition Planner
Computer Program.

It's hard to make sure that you and your family are getting the right balance of vitamins, minerals, proteins, carbohydrates, and fats for good health and long life. It's particularly hard to know how your diet is doing over the long term.

The East Meets West Nutrition Planner is designed to make getting good nutrition over the long term easy.

The Nutrition Planner is a computer program that calculates and stores not only the calories, but all the key nutrients for good health.

With it, you can determine the nutritional value of one meal or save and keep track of the nutritional value of your meals over a period of weeks, months, or years. You can readily identify what specific vitamins and minerals your diet lacks, and whether fat or salt may be in excess. You can follow your progress to a healthier diet and make corrections along the way.

The Nutrition Planner contains a large data base of both Japanese and Western foods. You just record what

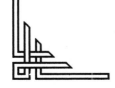

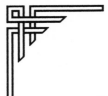
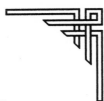

you've eaten. The computer does all the calculations and record keeping for you.

You can add new food items to the data base. The Nutrition Planner will learn and save the nutritional values for new recipes you give it.

Save the personal meal history of an unlimited number of individuals. Your whole family can benefit.

As of June 1989, the East Meets West Nutrition Planner is available only for IBM PC and compatible computers with 512K RAM and at least one floppy drive. The program can be copied to hard disk for greater ease of use.

Ask your local bookseller for the East Meets West Nutrition Planner or order directly from Ishi Press by sending $49.95 plus $3 shipping and handling to

Ishi Press International
1400 North Shoreline Boulevard, Bldg. A-7
Mountain View, CA 94043

Be sure to specify 5-1/4" or 3-1/2" diskette.

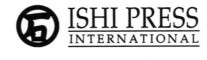

Start planning a
healthier diet today!

ISHI PRESS
INTERNATIONAL

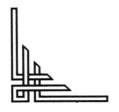
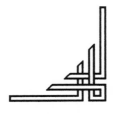